Health and Medicine
in the Catholic Tradition

Health/Medicine and the Faith Traditions

Edited by Martin E. Marty and Kenneth L. Vaux

Health/Medicine and the Faith Traditions
explores the ways in which major religions
relate to the questions of human well-being.
It issues from Project Ten,
an international program of the
Lutheran General Health Care System
in Park Ridge, Illinois.

Health and Medicine in the Catholic Tradition

TRADITION IN TRANSITION

Richard A. McCormick

Crossroad · New York

1985
The Crossroad Publishing Company
370 Lexington Ave, New York, N.Y. 10017

Library of Congress Cataloging in Publication Data
McCormick, Richard A.
Health and medicine in the Catholic tradition.
(Health/medicine and the faith traditions)
1. Medical ethics.   2. Medicine—Religious aspects—
Catholic Church.   3. Catholic Church—Doctrines.
I. Title.   II. Series.
R725.5.M39   1984   241'.642   84-21395
ISBN 0-8245-0661-8

For Phil and Barb
in lieu of counting the ways

Contents

Foreword

Try to think of a much more important topic than the one Father Mc-Cormick takes up here. G. K. Chesterton was once asked what he wanted out of the Church, and put it simply, "To get rid of my sins!" Since all Church people have, know they have, or should know they have plenty of sins that need good riddance, their agenda might well take priority over McCormick's. Give him another day and another assignment, he could no doubt write on that one. Let's just bracket that agenda for the moment and ask what is left over. Now it is hard to think of a topic much more important than one which asks and shows something about how to pursue bodily health and how to conceive what is good or bad in respect to persons in respect to such a theme.

The non-Catholic has much at stake here, too. For one thing, the Catholic tradition is embodied by several hundred million world citizens. What they think about one aspect of this topic, population planning and birth control, will have enormous consequences for the world's future. What they think about justice, about providing for health care, about care for the body, about finding meaning when suffering and death occur—as they must, and do, to all—will affect not only those hundreds of millions, but other Christians, other religious people, other people, as well. In other words, non-Catholics share ecumenical space with Catholics and had better understand them. Non-Catholics would do well to see what in this tradition might serve them well, and engage in dialogue or perform raids on the tradition for their own well-being.

A second reason for people to extend curiosity to Catholicism is the fact that it has such a rich if sometimes troubling tradition. Many institutions of mercy and healing in our cultures were invented by Catholic Christians in both the Middle Ages and the subsequent and still emerging modern world. To this day, hundreds of hospitals have the word "St." so-and-so chipped in concrete above the door, embossed in letterheads, and, through at least the intentions of those responsible, somehow coloring what goes on in the clinics. When citizens debate aspects of health care or medical ethics, they bump into Catholic declaration and practice. It would be foolish to come on the scene of medical ethical debates or the politics of health care without becoming aware of what the Catholic tradition has been and is today.

Now, the Catholic tradition does not have health and medicine to itself in a world we often call secular or pluralistic. This book is part of a series in which scholars will articulate aspects of the Muslim, Jewish, Hindu, and other traditions. Closer to (Catholic) home, two representations of "traditional" non-Roman Catholic lineages have already appeared. These deal with Lutheran and Reformed and thus with much of Protestant Christianity.

As an author of one of those books, I have learned how different it is to deal with such traditions, how contrasting is McCormick's assignment and fulfillment of his task. Catholicism has a pope, a magisterium, a defined pattern of authority. John Courtney Murray used to say that it took up space in the world in articulated and visible ways, so it was a Thing. No one can talk about the tradition without reckoning with its popes, its formal teaching authority. Not so in Protestantism, which has confessions but which looks as if it has only chaos. Kenneth Vaux and I more or less had to invent —look it up, invent, in the dictionary, means discover as well as fabricate— these traditions. McCormick has to confront his, with full knowledge that people have vested interests in saying that it is exactly this, or that.

His hazard would be to deal with the complexity of this tradition in such a way as to generate the chaos that Vaux and I set out to overcome in our own. He succeeds in doing this by focusing on a text, which makes up chapter 1. By concentrating on "Ethical Guidelines for Catholic Health Care Institutions," he has a definable and authoritative document to direct him. The reader gets confidence at once that the agenda is not private, idiosyncratic, set for tendentious purposes. This is what one must talk about if one wants to deal with the Catholic tradition today.

One can do many things with texts. It is possible to treat them purely historically. To do so in this case would have meant not writing a medium-sized book but a large-sized shelf or a small-sized library full of books. McCormick gets to the Catholic world behind the text only enough to help contemporary readers find their way and walk with some confidence. If one wishes to speak about a tradition in transition, it is necessary to know something of what that tradition is. Second, one can deal with the literary dimensions, the character of a text. McCormick must, but he is not a literary critic introducing us to the politics of text-preparation, the structure of the text, its modes of logic and rhetoric.

This book deals with a third use one can make of texts. They project a world, they push readers onto horizons they might otherwise not have explored, toward positions and ways of being that they might otherwise have overlooked. In that sense, this argument has a great deal to do with what lies ahead of Catholics and of non-Catholics who share a Catholic world. McCormick invites the reader to participate in a "transition," with all its fateful prospects and consequences.

When a relatively intact tradition is in transition, there is no helpful way to discuss it without taking some sort of stand. McCormick could have chosen either of two simple ways. He could have been a muckraker or a devastator, a person of but not at home with the Catholic tradition, who blasts away at its inconsistencies, shortcomings, and follies. Such "prophetic" works might have their place if they are written with a reformist intent by people who have the credentials. Such demolition is easy to do with any tradition, because, while its claims may be located in divine revelation, its custodianship is human, and history impinges on it at all points, thus subjecting it to potential devastation by those who lack empathy to go with their pride and, sometimes, their skills.

The other unhelpful way would have been to come on as a custodian of the custodians, who would exempt the tradition from critical scrutiny at all. McCormick theoretically could have been the keeper of the lock at the Catholic Museum, the duster of the antique-shop cases, the protector of antiquities. Yes, he could have been so theoretically, but not practically. His whole career has been given over to opening up the Catholic treasury, trying out its artifacts and achievements in the contemporary world, risking its values in a world that might need them more than it knows.

So he chose "the extreme middle," which is a good choice if you do not mind being shot at from all sides. Yet "extreme middle" need not and here does not mean a position which seeks mere balance, judicious stepping over land-mined territory, timid refusal to take a stand. This sort of middle is a bit like the kind Pascal talks about somewhere. It sets out to incorporate something of what is asserted in the strong truths of "yes" and "no" alike, and then to be strong in its own truths. McCormick does this with such respect for tradition and modernity, Catholicism and its context, authoritative teacher and questioner, that he might well make his points and proposals without alienating people from other kinds of extremes in the Church or without.

One hopes. One hopes that this voice of scholarship, fidelity, and care will through this book, as it has through previous writings, find a hearing. It would be a waste of time for readers to pick up a book on the Catholic tradition and find it unrepresentative of the concerns of that tradition. It would be an equal waste of time if the author discussed that tradition as if it were lead-encased and protected from a surrounding world, untouched by the history that so manifestly crowds in upon it at all times. It would be a waste of time if the "extreme middle" were bland, cautious. It is not a waste of time, but a very good investment of it, to read how McCormick uses some "Guidelines" to line out dimensions of a world that affect us all, and begins to guide us through it.

MARTIN E. MARTY

Introduction

The title of this volume is remarkably pretentious. It generates the impression that in these pages one will find an encyclopedic gathering of the history and reflection of a two-thousand-year-old believing community on a virtually inexhaustible topic ("being well"). Were such a volume to be written, it would have to be the result of a harmonious, multi-year conspiracy between exegetes, historians, patristic scholars, social scientists, philosophers, marriage experts, physicians, and theologians. There is only one Martin Marty in this world to constitute such a committee.

That being the case, it were well if I stated at the outset the limited ambitions of this volume. The term "Roman Catholic tradition" must be appropriately both narrowed and broadened. I have firsthand familiarity with and have been formed by a single cultural incarnation of that tradition. This incarnation can be described by a gathering of adjectives. For instance, one could begin by saying that it is American. That suggests in our time an immigrant church now come of age. Eugene Kennedy has described it as follows:

> The unlettered Catholics who came to the United States in the last century fashioned a way of life within the host Protestant culture that was tight, intellectually narrow, and wrapped in an invisible and largely impermeable membrane that resisted social osmosis with the rest of the country. It was also the most successful era of development in the history of the Roman Catholic Church. This Catholic structure defended itself proudly against doctrinal and moral compromise; it was, above all, obedient to the authority which was exercised for generations without any serious challenge by its bishops and clergy and other religious teachers. Immigrant Catholicism was, in fact, held together by the vigorous churchmen who retained their power over their flocks by exercising it regularly on an infinitely detailed category of behaviors, ranging from what the

1

faithful could eat on Fridays to what they could think or do in the inner-most chambers of their personal lives.[1]

Kennedy is suggesting above all that the immigrant Church was deeply authoritarian and paternalistic. Its major concern was the maintenance of the Catholic culture. With something like that in mind, Joseph Cardinal Bernardin recently stated that the contemporary American Catholic Church is poised between adolescence and adulthood.[2]

It is important to advert explicitly to this growth factor. If we do not, then the "Roman Catholic tradition" gets identified with one temporal manifestation of it, much as baseball should not be identified with the Chicago Cubs of 1922. Accidental dimensions are mistaken for the substance. Being stamped by an immigrant Church experience—and contemporary reactions to it—means that one has appropriated the tradition through this experience and must constantly struggle to be free of its limitations if one is to speak of *the* tradition.

By saying that the single incarnation is American, I mean also to suggest that it has been influenced by the typical characteristics of a Western in-dustrialized democracy. Technology, efficiency, and comfort are prized and maximized in such a society, and a believing community will undoubt-edly be touched, even tarnished, sometimes deeply, by the values dominant in the culture in which it resides. For that reason it is often difficult to dis-tinguish the tradition from its accompaniments. Thus the Church often mimics in her internal structures and life the characteristics of the culture in which she resides. It is no accident that the collegiality of bishops emerged in the Church at the very time the secular world and its institutions were turning to and relying on shared decisionmaking.

Another dimension of the American incarnation of the Catholic tradi-tion that should be stressed is the fact that it is both preconciliar and post-conciliar. This tradition was violently stirred and shaken by the Second Vatican Council. The Council altered the self-consciousness and the very model of the Church, changing it from pyramidal to concentric. The Cath-olic community is still in the process of adjustment, of assimilating and expressing in its life the profound *aggiornamento* initiated from 1962–65. It is no secret that some individuals find the work of the Council upsetting, distasteful, and destructive, and resist it with vigor. John XXIII referred to them as "prophets of gloom." Others, myself included, embrace it as the work of the Spirit. And even among those who embrace it, there are differ-ences about what it means. Furthermore, the American episcopacy has yet to achieve a maturity comparable to its size. A Canadian prelate—who shall remain unnamed—told me in 1980 that "your episcopal leadership is the most ultramontane in the world." All this suggests that the Roman Catholic tradition is in a state of flux, with dissonant voices claiming to possess it in its purest form.

In its twentieth-century, American incarnation, then, the Catholic tradition comes packaged in an immigrant community recently come of age (and therefore questioning the authority structure that was the vehicle of this tradition), hosted by a highly technological, industrial, and wealthy society (and therefore bearing the pluses and minuses of that society), and recently shaken to its roots by an ecumenical council whose efforts are still shaping the story of the Catholic community. This makes it especially difficult for those whom John Howard Yoder classifies as "agents of memory" to bring from the storehouse of their tradition memorable and identity-confirming acts of faithfulness and failure.[3] We must exert ourselves vigorously to shed the preconceptions of our own culture to get at *the* tradition. If we do not, we might easily confuse traditional ways of thinking and acting, which are often merely cultural appendages, with the religious tradition itself.

With these caveats in mind, I wish to state the limits within which I shall attempt to address the material of Project X. First, I will view the themes as a Catholic moral theologian. That means that I will be concerned with the normative dimension of our being and acting, with what we, as believers in Jesus Christ, *ought* to be and do (or not do). In this sense I will be concerned to lay out a moral tradition. Furthermore, it is only fair to warn the reader that every theologian shares in a tendency, is positioned somewhere along the liberal-conservative scale in her or his thought processes. Like many others, I mistrust those dichotomies and use them only because they are there and are current. Other terms are *open* and *closed*. However, it is unnecessarily provocative to refer to one's own stance as "open," implying that diverging perspectives are "closed." Therefore, in a spirit of happy abandon and Catholic irenicism, I shall suggest that the theological tendency at work here should be described as "the extreme middle."

Tradition, in its best theological sense, refers to a living reality. It is the ongoing appropriation of the Good News, the daily self-insertion into and reflection upon the narrative that has displayed God's gracious dealings with us. For this reason I propose to study the materials of Project X from a contemporary Catholic consciousness. I say "a" consciousness, because there are many personal and cultural appropriations of God's word in Christ and its implications for our behavior. So rich are the *magnalia Dei*, and so richly various their assimilations, that it would be presumptuous, and eventually idolatrous, to narrow them to "a" contemporary Catholic consciousness. "There are many mansions in my father's house."

The word *contemporary* must also be stressed. A living tradition includes the formative effect of the past. It is instructed by the past, but *pace* some reactionary Catholics, not paralyzed by it. I say this because there are still very many people who understand tradition exclusively as the past authoritative formulation of it. They get locked into words and into the limited historical consciousness that produced them in a way that deadens tradition and virtually invalidates contemporary experience and reflection.

This ossifying process has its roots in many human propensities (for example, attitudes toward authority). But regardless of its source, it is always characterized by a verbal and conceptual rigidity that fails to distinguish the substance of our convictions from their formulations. In his speech opening Vatican II, John XXIII noted that "the substance of the ancient doctrine of the deposit of faith is one thing, and the way in which it is presented is another."[4] This important distinction was reported in "The Pastoral Constitution on the Church in the Modern World." Our formulations are necessarily the product of a limited grasp of reality, of historically conditioned attitudes, of limited philosophical concepts and language. At a given time in history they are only more or less adequate. Our personal and communal task is constantly to purify these formulations, to bring them closer to the abiding substance of our religious or moral concern.

In this sense the word contemporary suggests that Catholic tradition is always innovative and, in a sense, always in flux. In its task of "formation of consciousness,"[5] it takes seriously the findings of human experience and human sciences. Its method is necessarily inductive. That means that it will at times necessarily say things that were not said before, and even modify things that were said before. It will not hesitate to be exploratory and tentative. (That is why the subtitle of this volume is *Tradition in Transition*.)

I want to emphasize this exploratory quality by appeal to the history of Catholic social teaching. This teaching developed roughly in three stages. The Encyclical *Rerum novarum* represents the first stage. It was dominated by "Christian philosophy" and a rigidly deductive method. This had two shortcomings. First, it left no room for the relevance of the social sciences. Second, and as a consequence, doctrinal elaboration was seen as an exclusively hierarchical task, laypersons being merely "faithful executors."

The second stage covers the pontificates of Pius XI and Pius XII and might be called the stage of "social doctrine." Indeed, *Quadragesimo anno* (authored in solitary splendor by Oswald von Nell-Breuning, S.J.) used this term for the first time. It referred to an organic corpus of universal principles still rigidly deduced from social ethics and constituted a kind of third way between liberalism and socialism. However, there is a greater emphasis on the historical moment and applications of principles to practice, hence the beginnings of a reevaluation of the place of laypersons in the process. Pius XI distinguished "unchanged and unchangeable doctrine" from social action, this latter being the competence of laypersons.

The third stage began with John XXIII. John moved from the deductive to the inductive method, his point of departure being the "historical moment" to be viewed in light of the Gospel. This led to a complete reevaluation of the place of laypersons vis-à-vis social teachings, a reevaluation completed by Vatican II. Laypersons do not simply apply the Church's social teaching; they must share in its very construction.

The novelty of this third stage is clear in the fact that the social teaching of the Church no longer refers to an immutable corpus of doctrine. Even the term "social doctrine" has fallen into disuse and is reserved for the period from Leo XIII to John XXIII. It is also clear in the new emphasis on the responsibility of the Christian community in the elaboration and application of the Church's social teaching, an emphasis most completely stated at Puebla (n. 473), the 1979 meeting of the Latin American bishops.

This interesting chronicle suggests a question: Has such a development occurred in the area of the Church's approach to the issues comprised under Project X? The answer is rather clearly no. Perhaps the question were better worded as follows: Should not such a development occur in the approach to these other questions? If a clearly deductive method, one that left little room for the sciences and lay experience, prevailed in the elaboration of social teaching, it is reasonable to think that the same thing occurred in familial, medical, and sexual morality. And if this method has evolved and changed during the pontificates of John XXIII, Paul VI, and John Paul II, it is reasonable to think that the same thing ought to happen in all areas of Catholic teaching. Yet two things seem clear about the Church's teaching on sexual, medical, and familial morality. First, earlier popes are invariably cited for their conclusions, not simply their systematic method. In other words, the teaching office of the Church more readily recognizes in the social sphere the factors that induce change than it does in the medical-familial-sexual sphere. Second, the sciences and lay experience remain marginal factors in the continuing reflection of the Church on familial, medical, and sexual matters.

I mention this at the outset because anyone attempting to unpack the Catholic tradition on well-being in a way that represents a *contemporary Catholic consciousness* of it must necessarily deal with factors still relegated to the marginal in some official methods and conclusions. It must deal with the groping developments and hypotheses that will be tomorrow's accepted orthodoxies and practices. This may lead some to wonder how something can be Catholic and yet not be found in official formulations of the tradition. To them I suggest that the term *the Catholic tradition* is a very broad one that includes far more than so-called official teaching. After all, Vatican II could only authenticate the teaching on religious liberty because it saw it as correct. That "seeing as correct" was a process. In its most inclusive sense the Catholic tradition can be understood as "the Catholic outlook on things," the Catholic way of conversing about and solving a problem. Within such an understanding of tradition there is even room for disagreement among Catholics, all of whom could legitimately claim they are working out of and representing the tradition. Whatever the case, such an understanding will be the backdrop against which this volume will develop its more concrete themes.

There are many ways of developing the themes of Project X. I will do it via a commentary on a document dealing with health and medicine in the Catholic setting. This document, "Ethical Guidelines for Catholic Health Care Institutions," was developed privately over a two-year period by a group of Catholic theologians, ethicists, and health care personnel. Their effort was generated by the suggestion in the introduction to "Ethical and Religious Directives for Catholic Health Facilities" (USCC, 1971) that the directives would need revision in light of scientific and theological development. The draft of the Guidelines used here has no official status. The Guidelines were neither commissioned nor approved by ecclesiastical authorities. Indeed, they might very well induce episcopal frowns and some crozier-thumping here and there. However, the authors of the draft inform me that broad consultation with people in the clinical setting involved in developing the Guidelines has revealed great support and approval of them. Thus they can lay claim to representing *a* contemporary Catholic consciousness.

It is my hope that the Guidelines will function as a prism through which the reader may be able to discern the substantial concerns of the Catholic tradition in health and medicine. Not all of the themes of Project X are explicitly addressed in the Guidelines. Furthermore, the Guidelines address subjects that would fit only uncomfortably under Project X. Yet there is sufficient overlap to hope that the essential purpose of Project X can be achieved by looking at the Guidelines. To this end, chapter 1 will simply present the Guidelines. Subsequent chapters will single out those of them that seem particularly suited to raise the issues of Project X. However, even those that are not the subject of explicit commentary will, I believe, serve the purpose of reflecting a contemporary Catholic consciousness.

· 1 ·

"Ethical Guidelines for Catholic Health Care Institutions"

INTRODUCTION

A. The Church's mission is to reveal and mediate the healing redemptive love of Jesus Christ in the world. Catholic health care institutions exist to be a visible expression of this mission. They should powerfully embody the Church's commitment to promote health and wholeness and to extend Christ's healing love to people whose lives have been disrupted by sickness, injury, or death.

B. Health includes the integration of the spiritual, the physical, and the psycho-social in every human person. Furthermore, the patient is an integrated whole, sometimes an individual, but often a family, a parent bonded with child, or a community. Catholic health care institutions affirm the centrality of the patient in the health care decisionmaking process. Moreover, the significant moral community surrounding the patient should provide support, counsel, and guidance in the decision-making process. The health care institution, as an extension of the religious and moral community of the patient, stands committed to provide compassionate support for the pursuit of the welfare and integrity of the patient.

C. In light of this broad notion of their mission, Catholic health care institutions ought to give sensitive care to the whole person, spiritual care as well as care for physical and psycho-social needs. Thus, pastoral care personnel have an indispensable role in the health care ministry.

D. If Catholic health care institutions are to achieve fully their mission, it is essential that all persons who work in them be aware of their respon-

8

sibility to contribute to an environment that will support and sustain loving care and respect for personal dignity. Those responsible for the governance of the institution have a special responsibility to foster awareness of the institution's primary reason for existence: to bring Christ's healing comfort and power to all.

E. From what has been said, it is clear that the Catholic health care institution exists to care. However, the best way to care in particular circumstances is not always perfectly clear, since values often come into conflict with one another. For help and guidance in resolving these conflicts, no source of moral knowledge should be neglected. Sources include: the experience of the health care and larger Christian communities, the local bishop, moral theologians and Church documents. In moral questions debated by moral theologians in the Church, Catholic tradition upholds the liberty to follow opinions which seem more in conformity with standards of good health care.

F. There are always conflicts and strains between individual needs and societal needs. These include the socio-political problems of health care delivery; the problems of a just system of health care. The solution of these larger public policy problems will deeply influence the shape of individual ethical decisions. Catholic institutions ought to be aware of this dimension of the problem of health care and attempt to play a significant role in its resolution. To do so effectively, Catholic institutions should recall that they have been and are, not only the channels that extend loving care to those in need; they have also been and are the bearers of our cultural distortions and injustices.

G. The following Guidelines are offered as a help to individuals, committees, and institutions toward fulfillment of their mission. The purpose of these Guidelines is to assist good ethical reflection and thus, good decisionmaking. They cannot replace individual conscience or personal and institutional responsibility. In fact, to remain contemporary and adequate to the constant developments in health care delivery, these Guidelines should be reviewed regularly.

GUIDELINES

1. Health care is a collaborative effort of the patient and skilled persons who share responsibility for the overall good of the patient. Policies and practices should support this collaborative effort, especially the

type of communication which prevents any member of the health care team from dominating others.

2. All personnel have a specific personal contribution to make to the spirit of the health care institution. This spirit should support dedicated care of the sick and sensitivity to the needs and concerns of everyone in the institution.

3. The administrative team, particularly the CEO, has a special responsibility to promote an atmosphere characterized by collaboration and mutual respect. To this end, all policies and practices should be reviewed regularly.

4. A health care institution relates to United States society and culture in significant ways:
   a) it can be seen as a microcosm of the larger society and its value priorities;
   b) it has strong bonds of interdependence with major dimensions of this society: legal, economic, technological, political, professional. In all of these societal relationships, institutions are presented with challenges regarding justice. Responses to these challenges should be shaped by the social teachings of the Church.

5. The employer/employee relationship demands particular attention. A just structure in this relationship calls for fairness and mutual accountability. Only in this way will the health care institution become a model of the justice it recommends to the broader society.

6. Independent practitioners are an important part of the health care institution's community. They are, then, accountable for the same standards of justice as are the salaried employees.

7. Concern for justice means that the health care institution will also turn outward to meet the needs of the underserved and the poor and do everything possible to influence public policy in this direction.

8. The health care institution should take seriously its responsibility to work for an equitable distribution of health care resources, both within the institution and in society as a whole. This includes involvement in areas of law and public policy.

9. Minority races have suffered deeply at the hands of our society. The same is often true in Catholic health care institutions, both with regard to employees and patients. Catholic institutions should play a

leading and aggressive role in redressing this imbalance, especially with regard to opportunities for advancement and respect for the dignity of patients.

10. A similar justice concern about the welfare of women—both patients and employees—should characterize a Catholic health care institution. Women and men should be afforded the same respect and consideration with regard to diagnoses and treatment. Women employees should have equal opportunity for employment and career development, and their work should be fairly compensated, i.e., in accord with the principle of equal pay for work of equal value.

11. The patient is the primary decisionmaker in all choices regarding health and treatment. This means that he or she is the first decisonmaker, the one who is presumed to make initial choices, based on his or her beliefs and values. Other secondary decisionmakers also have responsibilities. When the patient is legally incompetent or otherwise unable to take the initiative, an agent for the patient—normally the next of kin unless the patient has previously designated someone else or the next of kin is disqualified—has the responsibility to try to determine what the patient would have chosen, or, if that is impossible, what is in the patient's best interest.

    Health care professionals are also secondary decisionmakers, with responsibility to provide aid and care for the patient to the extent it is consistent with their own beliefs and values. Hospital policies and practices must recognize this set of responsibilities. Health care professionals are responsible for giving sufficient information and for providing adequate support to the patient to enable her/him to make knowledgeable decisions about appropriate care. It should be recognized that assistance in the decisionmaking process is an essential part of health care. Informed consent policies and documents should be geared to enhancing patient autonomy and protection, never primarily to protecting hospitals and health care workers from litigation.

12. Respect for persons implies respect for their privacy. At a time of computerized information and increasing impersonalization in the delivery of service, special attention to the rights of confidentiality is needed. Personnel should be aware of the ways in which confidentiality and privacy are violated, e.g., conversation in public places, access to patients' charts by unauthorized persons.

13. With increasing technology and specialization, the chances of deper-

sonalized care are increased. Catholic health care institutions should be especially sensitive to the rights of patients to be treated with respect, dignity, and personal attention.

14. Health care institutions are involved in aiding spouses to implement their procreative choices. In performing this service they should encourage responsible parenthood, which includes an openness to children, the appropriate limitation of conception when called for, and proper care of existing children. The moral status of some of the means to responsible procreation and limitation of children is controverted in the Church today. Health care personnel should be aware of these controversies, and health care institutions should take them into account in formulating their policies.

15. Since all individual human life deserves respect and protection, every reasonable effort must be made to nourish, support, and protect life in the womb. Thus, abortion has been rejected by the Church in the vast majority of instances as a violation of the respect due to nascent life.

16. Victims of rape require a special sensitivity, respect, and support because of the tragic and unjust nature of the experience and the frequently biased interpretation of what has occurred. As with all patients, the rape victim is the primary decisionmaker, a fact that can be easily forgotten because of the trauma of the experience and the emergency nature of the care. This means that treatment options must be very carefully explained. These options have important moral dimensions, some of which (prevention of implantation) are the subject of controversy in the Church. Health care institutions should be aware of these discussions and devise their policies in the light of them. Finally, adequate treatment must also include appropriate followup and support.

17. Infants and children, who are particularly helpless and dependent on others, have special needs and an equal right to care and attention. They should never be subjects of nontherapeutic experimentation which risks harming them in any significant way. Insofar as possible, children and adolescents should be included in decisionmaking about the treatment of their diseases and injuries.

18. The problem of the newborn with disabilities is one of the most anguishing and difficult that Catholic institutions face. What is appropriate treatment must be determined by a balance of the benefit and

burden of the treatment for the newborn. Treatments should not be extended where they offer no reasonable hope of benefit, or when the benefit is so overwhelmed by the burden that it must be said to be minimal and dispensable. Medical and surgical corrective procedures which are readily performed for otherwise healthy children should not be denied to handicapped children, unless the physical or mental handicap is so devastating that the child would derive no benefit from correction. Whatever their condition, these infants should never be the subjects of nontherapeutic research which risks harming them in any significant way. Every possible effort should be made to offer them and their families support, affection, and compassion during their short lives.

19. Health care providers should respect the continuing right of older persons to bear primary responsibility for decisions regarding their care. Providers should also recognize and respond to the special issues related to the care of the older person, e.g., privacy, sexuality, grieving, interaction of diseases; and coping with loss, progressive limitation, and depression.

20. Human suffering and death are an inescapable part of human life. However, through his own suffering and death Jesus has taught us that suffering and dying can be a means of inner transformation to deeper life as well as a redemptive prayer for others. Health care personnel should be trained and available to help patients find meaning in their experience of suffering and dying.

21. Though suffering and death are realities that cannot be eliminated, appropriate means should be taken to reduce suffering and preserve life. What means are appropriate is determined by a due proportion between the burden and the benefit of the treatment to the patient. If the treatment would only secure a precarious and burdensome prolongation of life, it may be refused by the patient or the family on behalf of the patient. Medications and other therapies whose purpose is to alleviate pain may be given as needed, with the consent of the patient or his or her agent, even if a side effect is the shortening of life. A person who is dying presents the health care team with one of its greatest challenges and opportunities. It is the challenge and opportunity to be with the dying and the family in a way which reproduces and mediates the fullest and final sense of Christ's healing love. Any medical treatment at this critical point must aim not at simply prolonging life, but at reducing the human diminishments of the dying process, maximizing the values the patient treasured in life, and bringing comfort.

22. As health care becomes more and more complex, there is a greater need for institution-wide deliberation on the ethical dimensions of decisions. One method of addressing this need is through committees which deal specifically with ethical and moral concerns. These committees do not relieve other individuals and groups of responsibility for ethical and moral reflection. They can, however, assist in good conscience formation by helping patients and other decisionmakers to identify values in conflict and by helping them to weigh all the elements and consequences of proposed personal and institutional decisions. These committees should represent a wide variety of backgrounds and expertise and should be educated in the processes of ethical decision-making.

·2·

Well-Being

The first four paragraphs of the "Ethical Guidelines for Catholic Health Care Institutions" represent a mission statement. That mission statement could be elaborated as follows.

There is a principle in Catholic moral theology known as the "principle of totality." It is shorthand for the moral legitimacy of removing or curtailing a function or an organ for the good of the whole person (thus the word *totality*). It was first called by this name in 1952, by Pius XII.[1] But the underlying idea is not new. Saint Thomas employed it to show why a diseased member could be sacrificed. Later Catholic theologians used it to justify even the excision of a healthy member.

In 1952, Pius XII referred to "the good of [a person's] being as a whole." Subsequent theological discussions have led to a virtual unanimity that what is meant by the principle of totality is the "total good of the person." It is the "total good of the person" that health care seeks, whether it be through surgery, spiritual counseling, care of the dying, psychotherapy, or anesthesia. Indeed, in a general sense, this "total good" is the ultimate aim of every human activity, but in the field of health care the phrase comes readily to Catholic lips. It is, I would think, identical in general content with the notion of well-being. Likewise, the term *healing* is also a rich and complex one. It cannot be restricted to an excision or an injection. It encompasses the "total good of the person."

What is included under that term? Vatican II asserted that the "moral aspect of any procedure . . . must be determined by objective standards which are based on the nature of the person and the person's acts."[2] The official commentary on this wording noted two things: that in the expression there is formulated a general principle that applies to all human actions, and that the choice of this expression means that "human activity must be judged insofar as it refers to the human person integrally and adequately considered" (*personam humanam integre et adequate considerandam*).[3]

Louis Janssens, building on the anthropology of Vatican II, suggests very helpfully that this phrase refers to the human person in all his or her essential aspects or dimensions.[4] He lists eight such aspects, the first being that the human person is a *subject* (normally called to consciousness, to act according to conscience, in freedom and in a responsible way). Christian revelation deepens our understanding of this subjectivity by stressing that each person is created in God's image (*Gaudium et spes*, 12, 17, 24, 29, 33, 37), is redeemed from his or her sinful situation by Jesus Christ (13, 22, 37), and is called to overcome death and share in God's kingdom (18, 21, 39, 45, 72, 93).

Second, the person is a bodily subject (14). Corporeality is essential to, and therefore shares in the excellence and dignity of, the human person. The Council noted that "the sexual characteristics of persons and the human faculty of reproduction wonderfully exceed the dispositions of lower forms of life" (51). This is true of all human activity.

Third, our body, as corporeal, forms a part of the material world. Thus we are beings-in-the-world whose challenge is to transform the natural milieu into a cultural one (56–62). "For the person, created in God's image, received a mandate to subject to himself or herself the earth and all that it contains and to govern the world with justice and holiness"(34). Thus, "they can justly consider that by their labor they are unfolding the Creator's work" (34). This has particular relevance to modern science and technology. Vatican II noted that "technology is now transforming the face of the earth and is already trying to master outer space"(5). In spite of its impressive achievements technological advance is frequently ambiguous. That is, it has positive and negative aspects and occasionally the negative effects outweigh its positive results (as in the case of pesticides that are carcinogenic). Notwithstanding the ambiguity of technology, Christianity remains basically optimistic about it. As Saint Thomas said, "We are sharers in God's providence by providing for ourselves and others."[5] God committed the natural order to us as intelligent and creative persons. In this sense, he is not only the creator of the natural order, but the enabler of our potentialities through our innovative interventions.

Fourth, human beings are essentially interpersonal. We grow and mature as subjects in essential interdependence on each other: only in relationship to a Thou does one become an I. We confer upon each other in relationship the capacity to take fuller possession of our humanity, to grow in the fullness of what we are. "For by their innermost nature persons are social beings, and unless they relate themselves to others, they can neither live nor develop their potential" (12). The "primary form" of interpersonal communion is the man-woman companionship, and its paradigmatic form is marriage.

Fifth, human persons must live in social groups with appropriate structures and institutions. Our structures and institutions must be worthy of persons and must reinforce their essential human characteristics (freedom, intelligence, conscience, etc.) and promote their growth. For this reason, Vatican II rejected a merely individualistic ethic and insisted that our responsibilities as persons extend to laws and institutions that support our lives within social groups (30).

Sixth, human persons are called to know and worship God in all that they do. This God-relationship is the most profound and ultimate aspect of the person. God is the source and destiny of the human person, and this relationship relativizes every other temporal good or evil.

Seventh, human persons are historical beings. The person matures through stages, each with specific challenges and possibilities. Furthermore, persons live in social groups that have their own cultural history and development. This means that a morality centered on the human person is a dynamic one. Vatican II duly noted this when it reminded us that "the human race has passed from a rather static concept of reality to a more dynamic, evolutionary one" (5). In adapting to the historicity of the person, a balanced wisdom is required, one that seeks a middle ground between uncritical enthusiasm and nostalgic condemnation. It is this latter that is the special danger of a community guided by an authoritative magisterium. As Janssens notes: "History itself testifies to so many mistakes which human beings later had to admit or ignore because they had too quickly condemned what was new without allowing for the *experience*, the time or the opportunity to work out whether or not something was worthy of human beings."[6] Vaccination against smallpox is a good example. In 1829 Leo XII declared, "Whoever allows himself to be vaccinated ceases to be a child of God. Smallpox is a judgment of God, the vaccination is a challenge toward heaven."[7]

Eighth, human persons, while unique and original, are fundamentally equal. Actions, practices, and institutions that implicitly deny or undermine this equality will not survive the scrutiny of a person-centered ethic.

In summary, when the person is "integrally and adequately considered," all of these essential dimensions must be taken into account: the person *in himself or herself* (1, 2) and in *his or her relations* (openness to the world, to others, to social groups, to God [3, 4, 5, 6]). Actions that promote the person adequately considered in this way are morally right; those that attack or undermine the person are morally wrong.

As Janssens insists, the Council continuously pointed out that the moral criterion is the *whole person*. For instance:

The *human person* deserves to be preserved; human society deserves to be renewed. Hence the pivotal point of our total presentation will be the person himself or herself, whole and entire, body and soul, heart and conscience, mind and will.[8]

Often refusing to acknowledge God as their beginning, human beings have disrupted also their *proper relationship to their own ultimate goal.* At the same time they became *out of harmony with themselves, with others, and with all created things.*[9]

It remains each person's duty to preserve a view of the *whole person*, a view in which the value of *intellect, will, conscience, and fraternity* are preeminent. These values are all rooted in God the Creator and have been wonderfully restored and elevated in Christ.[10]

In the socioeconomic realm, too, the *dignity and total vocation of the human person* must be honored and admired along with the *welfare of society as a whole.*[11]

The fundamental purpose of this productivity [of goods in agriculture and industry] must not be the mere multiplication of products. It must not be profit or domination. Rather it must be the service of human beings, and indeed of the whole person, viewed in terms of their material needs and the demands of their intellectual, moral, spiritual, and religious life. And when we say person, we mean *every person whatsoever and every group of persons* of whatever race and from whatever part of the world.[12]

I have emphasized the centrality of the person—the whole person, including the communities and institutions around the person—for several reasons. First, over the centuries this insight was neglected, and isolated aspects of the person, particularly biological aspects, became normative. One can see this in the writings of F. Hürth, S.J., who was very influential in the pontificate of Pius XII. It is a known fact that Hürth was largely responsible for the major writings of Pius XII on sexual and medical questions. Hürth regarded procreativity as the exclusive primary finality of human sexuality. For him, this was "the intention of nature inscribed in the organs and their function" ("*la volonté de la nature inscrite dans les organes et leur function*").[13] Thus artificial insemination by the husband was to be excluded as against nature—and indeed Pius XII did formally condemn it on three occasions.

At one point in his analysis of the marriage act Hürth states:

Our whole argument proves not only that nature has determined the means for human beings by which they are capable of serving the species, but also that they may only serve it by this means, i.e., the natural marriage act. It would be absurd that nature determined the means for humans in every respect (anatomical, physiological, psychological) to place themselves at the service of the species and that it indicated the manner of acting to the smallest detail with an almost unbelievable efficiency in order to thus allow humans the right to choose their manner of acting as they please or to substitute another means for it which they had found themselves. Nature contains no such inner contradiction. Let me conclude: This analysis of the psychosomatic sexual apparatus demands that we say that our right to use the sexual organism, and especially the germ cells, is limited to the execution of the natural marriage act with all that prepares for, accompanies, and follows from it in a natural way.[14]

It is clear, then, that for Hürth the moral law and the biological law coincide. Indeed, Hürth states exactly that.

Human beings only have disposal of the use of their organs and their faculties with respect to the end which the Creator, in his formation of them, has intended. This end for humans then is both the biological law and the moral law, such that the latter obliges them to live according to the biological law.[15]

In such reasoning it is not the whole person that is central and normative, but the biology of the person.

The second reason for emphasizing the centrality of the person ("integrally and adequately understood") is that it becomes clear that a moral assessment of our actions must consider the *whole action*—external act, intention, circumstances, consequences—for each of its aspects has an effect upon the person.

The final reason for emphasizing the person is that this emphasis is essential to the notion of health and healing in the Catholic tradition. Thomas Clarke, S.J., points out that Jesus' exercise of power "is presented as *healing*, as *liberation*, as *restoration to wholeness*. The three models intertwine, in keeping with the biblical understanding of health as wholeness, and of sickness of any kind as subjection to the power of Satan."[16] As A. Oepke notes, "hardly another image impressed itself so deeply on early Christian tradition as that of Jesus as the great physician." [17] Clarke summarizes his reflection on the Gospels as follows:

The central thrust of this exercise of power is conceived as liberation from Satan, healing and restoration to health, and wholeness of human beings in the totality of their lives, physical and moral, social and institutional.[18]

As noted, paragraphs A, B, C, and D of the "Ethical Guidelines for Catholic Health Care Institutions" constitute a mission statement. Christ's love is described in A as "redemptive and healing," the latter being instrumental to the former. Just as the Church is the continuation of Christ's presence, the primordial sacrament (Rahner), so Catholic health care institutions find their raison d'être in being expressions of that healing and redemptive love. Once this is said, it is clear that health and healing have been given meanings far broader than the administration of technology and medicine to the body.

Paragraph A is undoubtedly the most important in the Guidelines. It tells Catholic health care institutions *why* (final cause) they exist and, in doing so, *how* they should exist. With the decline of religious vocations (most Catholic health facilities are operated by religious) and the increasing technology of health care, there has been something of an identity crisis in Catholic health care institutions. Questions often asked are: How do Catholic health care facilities differ from secular ones? Should they be continued under religious sponsorship? Would not the energies and personnel of the sponsoring religious body be better used elsewhere?

The answer to these questions given by the Guidelines is found in the term *visible expression*. Human beings are not disincarnate spirits. We are corporeal subjects. Furthermore, we are redeemed in Christ. We share the unspeakable life of God's love, his familyship—now mysteriously and inchoately, but nonetheless really. The Church, the extension of Christ's presence, is in the business of spreading this good news. To spread the good news means to do all those things that remind us of who we really are. We are reminded of our true worth by being treated in accordance with this dignity. It is axiomatic that we expand and become capable of love by being loved. Hence the Church's proclamation is necessarily action. The Church is in the health care apostolate because it is a most concrete and effective way of communicating to human beings their real worth—that is, the good news. For if the Church proclaims to people what they truly are here and now, yet does nothing about it, she literally does not mean what she says. Proclamation of the Gospel is by inner necessity concern for those to whom the Gospel is proclaimed. The Church's ethical action is an *anticipation* of the kingdom, and, as such, a proclamation of it. We need our "visible expressions" of who we are.

Walter Burghardt, S.J., sees the Catholic health apostolate as a form of service that empowers others to reach their human and Christian potential.

> You help an ailing member of Christ's body to realize his or her potential as a human person, as a Christian person. Sickness is not something out-

side of me. *I* am sick, not simply my head or my heart, my colon or my kidney. And it is on this rack, on this bed of pain, that I must work out my salvation. It is *I* to whom you minister: to my fears, to my feeling of help-lessness, my diminishment as a person. I am coming apart. I am not the whole person who once gloried in my flesh, in my lustiness, in my strength. I need the support of the body that has nourished me since my baptism— and at this moment *you* are that body in miniature. I need you, not simply to ease my pain, not primarily to make me *feel* better. I need you to work out my salvation with me. Not a pious lecture on Gethsemane and the cross; I know all that! Rather, the strength, the grace that comes to the heavy-burdened when I am surrounded by my special family, a genu-inely Christian family, a household of love.[19]

Paragraph B of the Guidelines is an attempt to define health in a very broad sense, as spiritual, physical, and psychosocial—healing involves all of these dimensions. Burghardt refers to "my special family" and B empha-sizes this by noting that the patient is an "integrated whole . . . often . . . bonded with . . . a community" and that the health care facility is an ex-tension of this "significant moral community."

Obviously, things do not always work out this way. Some patients have no moral community. Furthermore, medical, nursing, and paramedical personnel are often members of different faith communities and it is a bit of a stretch to see them as "an extension of the religious and moral commu-nity of the patient." But being a mission statement, B describes an ideal. Its meaning is that a health care institution should try to organize itself and behave as if it were an extension of the patient's religious and moral com-munity. It ought to respect and support the religious and moral values of the patient to the extent that this is possible. The patient should experience the health care institution as an extension of his or her community. It is in this sense that B insists that "Catholic health care institutions affirm the centrality of the patient in the health care decisionmaking process."

Paragraph C carries the implications of this broad notion of mission to the whole person a step farther by insisting that pastoral care personnel are essential to the health care ministry. There are several reasons for this em-phasis. First, there is the conviction that holistic health care must include spiritual ministration to the patient.

Second, pastoral-care departments are relatively new developments. In a recent survey conducted by Joseph Fichter, S.J., three-fourths of the hos-pitals responding had organized pastoral care departments.[20] In 1971, according to a Catholic Hospital Association survey, only one-fifth had pastoral care departments. Being relatively new additions to health care institutions, pastoral care departments still have to fight for recognition within these institutions. This is especially the case since these departments are often heavily staffed with women, especially religious sisters. Some people still resist the idea that religious women (or women generally) can perform tasks formerly reserved to male chaplains or ordained priests.

Third, in the past, chaplaincy work was often performed by priests who had no special training for this work. As Fichter noted, "Often they acted as spiritual director for the religious community of sisters operating the hospital and were appointed because they themselves needed medical attention, or had been found inadequate to fulfill other roles of the ordained ministry in parishes and mission."[21] This lack of training, and often of competence, generated attitudes and policies that are hard to change, even though today's pastoral care personnel are often well-trained and certified professionals.

The final, and perhaps most important, reason for stressing the essential role of pastoral care personnel is that too many physicians and surgeons seem not to recognize it and they continue to regard all others in the health care facility, including pastoral care personnel, as their subordinates.

Paragraph D moves beyond the pastoral care department and asserts that all persons in the health care institution have a responsibility for the environment that supports the mission of the institution. This is an attempt to hold up as an ideal the notion of the therapeutic community. William Kenney and Charles Ceronsky have noted that "if a Catholic health facility is to witness to Christian values today, it must do so through the services rendered and values expressed by its employees in their contacts with patients and fellow staff."[22] It is one thing to have a mission statement; it is another to carry it out *effectively*. This latter is achieved only under a twofold condition. First, all the employees must work toward the goal of providing an atmosphere of loving concern and competent caring. This is especially true of nurses, whose contacts in the institution are most far-reaching and whose dealings with patients are most intimate and knowledgeable. Catholic health care institutions have discovered that employees do not know much about the religious heritage of these institutions. This is a significant discovery, because the institutions' sisters have reasoned that as their numbers dwindle, lay employees will carry on the Catholic mission of charity begun by the sisters. And that will be difficult if employees know little about that mission. As Sister Agnes Marie says of Saint Charles Hospital in Oregon, Ohio, where she served from 1954 to 1981: "Sure, we had a values statement. But were our employees aware of it? We found they did not know much about the Sisters of Mercy or our tradition of caring."[23]

D refers to the responsibility of all to contribute to "an environment that will support and sustain loving care and respect for personal dignity." Those last four words may seem vague at first, but they become vivid in light of Dr. Lawrence K. Altman's description and indictment of hospital practices. Altman emphasizes the sense of deep embarrassment that can come over one in a hospital: "It's a kind of humiliation that seems to grow out of vulnerability, nakedness, of being handled, left exposed to be clinically peered at and examined like a grapegruit in a grocery."[24]

Some indignities, Altman noted, are unavoidable; others are not:

> The ill-fitting gowns that leave you standing in the hallway or x-ray department showing more of yourself than any passerby has a right to see; or the almost indescribably mortifying experience of being carried as an invalid from one treatment area to another by callous hospital workers, moving your body along as if it were being loaded on a ship by longshoremen; or being exhibited in a teaching hospital to groups of strangers who discuss you impersonally in your own presence, using language you don't understand; or revealing intimate details about your life history or finances in a crowded office where everyone can overhear.

Altman is quick to insist that it is not only physicians who are to blame.

> They are far outnumbered by nurses, clerks, secretaries, orderlies, elevator operators, janitors, and others. Too few medical centers train staff members to be more sensitive to patients' needs and to listen more carefully to their complaints.

The second condition necessary for effective mission is that "those responsible for the governance of the institution" create and promote the atmosphere in which this is possible. This is called a "special responsibility" to emphasize the facts that others are not exempt from it and that administrators do indeed have the capacity to "foster awareness of the institution's primary reason for existence." The problem, of course, is how to achieve this. There are dozens of things that can be done, from warm and imaginative ways of welcoming new patients to educating employees about the history and mission of the sponsoring religious body. However, D is concerned not with innovative details, but in focusing responsibility for them where it belongs. If this responsibility is not discharged vigorously and creatively, Catholic health care institutions will be identified largely by what they do not do (abortions and, with qualifications, sterilizations) rather than by what they do. As Sister Agnes Marie Bocs, executive director of the Mercy Health Care System in the Cincinnati Province put it:

"Most important . . . is whether we heal as Jesus did. That makes us more Catholic than the fact that we don't do abortions."[25]

Paragraphs A, B, C, and D, then, hold up a vision of health care wherein the patient-person as a whole (spiritual, physical, and psychosocial) is the focal point. From the Catholic point of view this means to "extend Christ's love" in the full biblical sense of health and healing. If this vision or purpose is absent, the "Catholic" health care facility becomes superfluous and the mission of the believing community in this area becomes fruitless. If the identification remains negative, not only will the institution fail in its major apostolic purpose, but even those negatives ("what they do not do") will have lost the heartbeat that supports them. In short, Catholic facilities must constantly ponder this question: "If you were indicted for being a Catholic hospital, would there be enough evidence to convict you?"

This means that "those responsible for the governance of the institution" must show a strong capacity for leadership. The notion of leadership is so important to the overall mission of the Catholic health care institution that it demands careful analysis. What can easily be forgotten is that leadership affects the "climates" in which we live and grow. "Climates" affect *whether* we grow as humans and Christians. By "climates" I refer to our manner of doing things, lifestyle, attitudes, and habits of action, reaction, and speech. These have a profound influence on how we think, feel, and behave. They seep through our pores and shape our decisions. The omnipresent danger is that corrosive values and priorities of a secular, material, and unbelieving world will infiltrate health care facilities and shape their policies.

Most people would concede that there is a crisis of leadership in the United States today, and, more narrowly, in the American Catholic Church. We suspect that politicians covet public office not for what they can do with it for us, but for the sake of power and its perquisites. There is a gnawing fear that some in the Church look to the pastorate, episcopate, and cardinalate as a reward. The heart of the crisis centers around the issues of authority and leadership. An analysis of authority and leadership and of the Christian notion of leadership may help health care institutions better realize their mission.

AUTHORITY AND LEADERSHIP

It is obvious that authority and leadership are closely related. I understand authority as the right to speak for, decide for, a particular group, to bind the members to the goals and methods of the group. It is the right to command and order. Leadership is the capacity to influence the behavior of a group toward some goal; it can be executive, administrative, or charismatic. Leadership, it is clear, is much broader than authority. There are many ways to influence conduct other than by command. One can command all day without being a leader.

Nonetheless, we are constantly tempted to identify the two notions—as though a badge made a good policeman, an M.D. a good physician, or a miter a good bishop, the robe the competent judge, the degree a creative theologian. When authority and leadership are simply identified in a group's day-to-day structures, a strange thing happens: leadership begins to disappear or shift locus. For the more one relies on mere office, the less one does those things required for real leadership. The steps that follow are predictable and quite human. First, actual leadership wanes. Second, as it does so, authority figures appeal all the more to their position, authority, and office. We hear appeals such as "your president," "your bishop," "your boss," "your father and mother." Finally, as actual authority weakens, the protest against authoritarianism grows. But this is not basically a protest. It is a hope. We submit to authority in the hope that it will become leadership. Authoritarianism is authority that has ceased to struggle to become leadership. Our resentment of mere authority reveals our desire for authority that struggles to become leadership.

There is a paradox in the identification of authority and leadership. The more authority is *factually* separate from leadership, the more authority figures identify them. Because they are not leaders, authority figures cling desperately to what they are—bearers of juridical authority. Conversely, the more authority and leadership are combined, the more they are distinguished and the less appeal there is to position. The hold on authority is more relaxed.

The tendency to identify leadership with office is a very human tendency. It is buried deep in the human mystery of the recoil before challenge, of the dread of loneliness, of the intolerance of insecurity. The true leader must survive all of these. Thus, for example, parents react to the exciting if frustrating challenges and inconsistencies of children with appeals to authority. Yet a man is not fully a father (leader) or a woman a mother by mere biological status, their "office." Priests can easily narrow their ministerial credentials to the oils of ordination. Yet ordination is a challenge to the ordained to grow to the fullness of his anointing, to become what he is. A teacher is not an effective teacher by rank or tenure. Yet too many teachers squelch questions or disagreements by appealing to their position or experience. This is the educator's way of confusing authority and leadership.

The careless identification of leadership with mere office yields two results. First, an independent value is attributed to office, formal authority, or credentials. But formal authority is a subordinate value. When it becomes independent (instead of serving others), it becomes that which is served, preserved, maintained, maximized. There is a predominant concern for the prerogatives of office, and a corresponding blindness to the goals it serves. Threats to authority are seen as threats to the faith. That is when "all the president's men" are born, whether in a family, a school, a church, a business, or a government. When mere authority is assigned an independent value, it is useless from the Christian point of view.

Second, we begin to experience the controlled group. Parents cease loving their children and begin controlling and dominating them. Teachers cease educating and begin controlling, using students for their own prestige. Bishops do not maximize the apostolic effectiveness of their priests; rather they "keep them in line." Politicians cease serving their constituents and begin manipulating them. Students begin playing a game rather than learning and attempting to grow. This is sad because playing a game is nearly always playing someone else's game.

The symptoms of control and the controlled group are well-known. In teaching, there is the dominance of the negative, the condemnatory, and the intolerance of pluralism. In administering there is oppressive centralization. There is avoidance of risk, conformism, "don't-rock-the-boat-ism." In policy planning there is waffling, fear of the fresh issue, enslavement to traditional phrases, anger at uncertainty. The use of power is secretive. Discussion is closed and draws on limited competence, usually those who agree in advance with the institutional position. The controlled are told what they may and may not do, not what they can achieve. They are reminded of the importance of a structure, not their own importance. They are constrained, not challenged, forbidden, not stimulated. All of these things can and do happen in families, businesses, universities, the Church, government—and in health care facilities.

There is an acceptable language that cloaks all of this: "national interest," "good of the country," "health of the country," "disturbance of the faithful," "my pastoral responsibilities." All of these have, of course, a legitimate meaning. But on the lips of the controller they only thinly disguise the priority of existing ways over the goals they serve, *my* ways over the growth of those committed to me.

The personality traits of the controlled are equally clear: fear, anxiety, joyless security, rejection of creative risk, growing apathy. In the Church there is a suffocating ultramontanism.

Giving an independent value to office or authority is a constant human temptation. Saint Paul saw it in the Galatian community. The Galatians fell back on the observance of the law and sought a sense of religious security from it. As Quentin Quesnell has observed:

> Religion has always offered this possibility to men to some extent. All organizations and institutions do it in some measure. But true Christianity, with its frightening message of faith and its constant demand for free faith given daily, given almost from moment to moment, deprives men of this support. A basic craving remains unsatisfied. An instinctive tendency of religious psychology continues to exert its drive; and the little flock of Christians begins to fall into the system of order, of law, of obedience, of institutionalization against which Paul warns so vigorously here.[26]

This is the temptation of Christians at all times. The simple identification of authority and leadership with all its results is a contemporary form of Galatianism.

A CHRISTIAN NOTION OF LEADERSHIP

It is regrettable that the phenomenon just described occurs in the Church and in Christianity in general. For we have in our roots and traditions an unmistakable picture of the basic element of true leadership. What is that element? In and beneath all forms of leadership (whether charismatic, executive, or administrative) one finds the release, stimulation, evocation, maximization of the potential of the individual. True leadership calls forth the best in those led. It liberates them into the fullness of their potential and most generally by moving minds and hearts.

Jesus' love is the paradigm here. It is effective. It empowers us, makes us "new creatures." It empowers us to love God in our neighbor. It is the source of our love for one another. So, too, our love for others, if it takes its shape from Jesus, should be empowerment. In other words, in Jesus, God confronts us to tell us who we are and what we may become, to enlarge our humanity, to create and deepen our capacity for the Godlife. He confronts us to mirror to us our true potential, and by mirroring to confer it. This conferring liberates us from those cultural, hereditary, and personal hangups and deformities that drain self-respect and stifle our growth.

Therefore, true leadership, if it builds on the example of Jesus, does not control. *It liberates.*

> A dispute also arose among them about which should be reckoned the greatest, but he said to them, "Among pagans it is the kings who lord it

over them, and those who have authority over them are given the title Benefactor. This must not happen with you. No; the greatest among you must behave as if he were the youngest, the leader as if he were the one who serves."[27]

You know that among the pagans their so-called rulers lord it over them, and their great men make their authority felt. This is not to happen among you. No; anyone who wants to become great among you must be your servant, and anyone who wants to be first among you must be slave to all. For the Son of Man himself did not come to be served but to serve, and to give his life as a ransom for many.[28]

How do we serve others? If we take Jesus seriously, it is precisely by liberating them into the fullness of their potential. For Jesus is God's empowerment of us. To serve, therefore, means to aid others in the move from self-distrust to self-esteem, from anxiety to peace, from emptiness and alienation to joyful hope, from the slavery of compromised secular value judgments to fearless Christian value judgments, from cringing securityism to the adventures of risk.

If to lead is to empower others into the fullness of their potential, then every office, every position, every reward, and every institution exists for this purpose. Thus the motto of the Christian leader might well be, "He must increase; I must decrease."

If this liberating mentality and atmosphere dominates us, we will experience its delightful results: security amid confusion, peace amid disagreement, unity amid pluralism, freedom amid regulation and law, loyalty amid dissent, and hope in a broken world.

In this atmosphere, the parent who punishes a child does so clearly because the punishment is an extension of his or her loving. The pope or bishop who commands, admonishes, and demands, does so clearly because he seeks the Christian good of the people.

In the end, therefore, office and leadership, though distinguished, should be factually conjoined. Those with position—any position—should be leaders. This is true if we do not succumb to a single notion of leadership —the charismatic. We are a hero-worshiping culture, the type that singles out charismatic types for the covers of *Time* and *Newsweek*. Hence charismatic leadership tends to shape our expectations and structure our criticism. Furthermore, our world is bureaucratized and institutionalized. Charismatic persons provide relief from sheer hugeness, facelessness, and impersonality. They confer on us a warm and welcome sense of the value of being human, distinct, and of worth. Thus charismatic leadership is more appealing than less spectacular forms. One thinks of John XXIII, John F. Kennedy, Martin Luther King, Dorothy Day, Helder Camara, and Mother Teresa.

But there are other types of leadership that challenge us little people in our ordinary lives. We can and must be leaders without being charismatic figures. It is here that most authority finds its contemporary challenge to become leadership. Authority will begin to coincide with leadership if it makes its overriding concern the releasing of the potential of others. And our most profound potential has been conferred on us in Jesus: a potential for the God-relationship, to love God in our neighbors. The most sublime form of leadership is expanding *that* potential.

As Christians, we should know all of this. If the Christian notion of leadership begins with the person of Christ, if his person shouts loudly of serving, if this service is liberating (empowering) us into our true potential, then is not leadership present whenever the true potentials of the group are released?

A bishop is a true leader when he makes it possible for the theologian to become a better theologian; a layperson to be a better Christian educator, parent, or businessperson; the priest to be a better apostolic instrument. He has conjoined authority and leadership because he uses authority to maximize the potential of others. The businessman whose day-to-day combining of quality with honesty inspires others to do the same is a true leader. He has conjoined position with leadership because he uses his position to empower others. Parents who entrust proportionate responsibility to their children and guide them into gradual self-possession are true leaders. They have conjoined position and leadership by using their status to liberate others.

In his book *Of Kennedys and Kings*, Harris Wofford describes a friend of mine as follows:

> Shriver was not a tidy administrator, but he was a great executive. He did not delegate powers through an orderly chain of command, but he empowered people. He released their energies, backed their efforts, and drew on their insights.[29]

That is what I mean by leadership. The form it will take for most of us will not be easy. It is humble, quiet, painstaking, often dreary and unsensational. It is full of risks and doubts. It is lacking in immediate satisfaction and public kudos. It is fairly bristling with sacrificial demands.

It is the parent who stands bleary-eyed and dog-tired over a sick child at

3 A.M. It is the teacher who fights through a batch of homework essays when he is dying to catch the last quarter of a football game. It is the young man and woman in love who struggle to protect each other when the whole world tells them to enjoy each other. It is the professional woman who files an exact expense account when no one is looking over her shoulder. It is all of these things that eventually empower others and therefore are the stuff of leadership. As a sage might put it: certain things must be caught rather than taught.

If "those responsible for the governance of the institution" do not aspire to be true leaders in this sense, the Catholic health care facility may as well close its doors.

THE DEPTH OF WELL-BEING

The term *healing* points to the term *health*. And when healing is said to concern "the patient-person as a whole," to "extend Christ's healing love," then, clearly, *health* includes well-being in all its dimensions. Therefore, the well-being that is the aim of healing necessarily includes and is described in light of a thoroughly Christian anthropology, our "being in Christ." In what follows, I will attempt to describe the transformative influence of the faith experience, to show the relativizing influences of the love command, and to relate these to health care. Only when this is done will we have some inkling of the enormity of the challenge contained in the Guidelines' mission statement. In this effort to outline a Catholic anthropology for health care, I shall call to witness several theological colleagues, especially Joseph Sittler, William F. May, Gerard Gilleman, S.J., and Enrico Chiavacci (the first two, interestingly enough, non-Catholic).

Let me begin with a statement of Johannes B. Metz: "Christ must always be thought of in such a way that he is never merely thought of."[30] Merely to "think of" Christ is to trivialize him, to reduce him to one more (among many) observable historical events, to an example of humane benevolence. For Christians, Jesus Christ is God's immanent presence, his love in the flesh. As William F. May puts it: "Jesus himself is the event in which the promises of God are fulfilled. He is the terrain, temple, and king, if you will, in which men may encounter God in his own person."[31]

Joseph Sittler has noted that the theme of the biblical narratives is God's "going out from himself in creative and redemptive action toward men."[32] Sittler refers to "God's relentless gift of himself," "the undeviating self-giving God," "the total self-giving of God," "God's undeviating will to restoration," the "history-involved assault of God upon man's sin," "the gracious assault of his deed in Christ." Jesus Christ is no less than God's self-giving deed.

The response of the believer to this person-revelation is the total commitment of the person known as faith. The term *faith* has had an uneven history in Christianity. Too often it has been tied to a pale propositional understanding of God's deed in Christ. Once again, Sittler:

> It is not possible to state too strongly that the life of the believer is for Paul the actual invasion of the total personality by the Christ-life. So pervasive and revolutionary is this displacement and bestowal that terms like influence, example, command, value are utterly incapable of even suggesting its power and its vitally recreating force.[33]

The believer's response to this specific, momentous, and supreme event of God's love is total and radical commitment. For the believer, Jesus Christ, the concrete enfleshment of God's love, becomes the meaning and *telos* of the world and of the self. God's self-disclosure in Jesus is at once the self-disclosure of ourselves and our world. "All things were made through him, and without him was not anything made that was made."[34] Nothing is intelligible without reference to God's deed in Christ. The response to this personal divine outpouring is not the dead "amen" of the bystander. It is a faith-response empowered by the very God who accomplished the redemptive and restorative deed in Jesus Christ and is utterly and totally transforming—so much so that Saint Paul must craft a new metaphor to articulate it. We are "new creatures," plain and simple. Faith is the empowered reception of God's stunning and aggressive love in Jesus. As theologian Walter Kasper summarizes it:

> Faith is not simply an intellectual act or an act of the will. It includes the whole man and every aspect of the human reality.... It embraces the whole of Christian existence, including hope and love, which can be seen as two ways in which faith is realized.[35]

This same point is underlined by Sittler when he notes that faith is the proper term "to point to the total commitment of the whole person which is required by the character of the revelation."[36]

Sittler has noted that "to be a Christian is to accept what God gives."[37] And what God gives is the going-out from himself in Jesus Christ. Something *has been done* to and for us and that something is Jesus. There is a prior action of God at once revelatory and response-engendering. Sittler correctly insists that the passive verb dominates the New Testament. "I love because I am loved; I know because I am known; I am of the Church, the body of Christ, because this body became my body; I can and must forgive because I have been forgiven."[38] This prior action of God is reflected in the Pauline "therefore" (*oun*) which states the entire grounding and meaning of the Christian ethic.

The Italian theologian Enrico Chiavacci puts it this way:

> In the New Testament the unique obligation of charity, which is the giving of self to God who is seen in one's neighbor, is grounded on the unique fact that God is charity. . . . "Walk in love *as* Christ has loved us and given himself" (Eph. 5:2). "*Therefore*, I exhort you brethren, through the mercy of God to offer yourselves. . ." (Rom. 12:2). The fact that God —in his manifestation as philanthropy—is love does not refer to further justification; it is the ultimate fact. The obligation to love is based only on God's love for us. . . . It is true . . . that in the "therefore" of Romans 12:1 we find the entire New Testament ethic.[39]

Here I want to make six points in a systematic way. First, as already noted, in Christian ethics God's self-disclosure in Jesus Christ as self-giving love allows no further justification. It is the absolutely ultimate fact. The acceptance of this fact into one's life (*fides qua*) is an absolutely originating and grounding experience.

Second, this belief in the God of Jesus Christ means that "Christ, perfect image of the Father, is already law and not only law-giver. He is already the categorical imperative and not just the font of ulterior and detailed imperatives."[40]

Third, this ultimate fact reveals a new basis or context for understanding the world. It gives it a new, Christocentric meaning. As a result of God's concrete act in the incarnation, "human life has available a new relation to God, a new light for seeing, a new fact and center for thinking, a new ground for forgiving and loving, a new context for acting in this world."[41]

Fourth, this "new fact and center for thinking" that is Jesus Christ finds its deepest meaning in the absoluteness and ultimacy of the God-relationship. The person of Jesus is testimony to the fact that "no effort of man to know himself, find himself, be himself, is a viable possibility outside the God-relationship."[42]

Fifth, this God-relationship is already shaped by God's prior act of self-giving in Jesus. "To believe in Jesus Christ, Son of God, is identical with believing that God—the absolute, the meaning—is total gift of self."[43] Therefore, the "active moment of faith takes place in the recognition that meaning is to give oneself, spend oneself, and live for others."[44] There is a German axiom that states: "Every gift constitutes an obligation" (*jede Gabe ist eine Aufgabe*). That is profoundly true here. The very gift of God in Jesus constitutes or shapes the response; thus it is proper to refer at once to "God's love-gift and command." The Christian moral life must be viewed as "a reenactment from below on the part of men of the shape of the revelatory drama of God's holy will in Jesus Christ."[45] In this sense, it is the "following of Christ." It is a recapitulation in the life of the believer of the "shape of the engendering deed," to use Sittler's phrase.

Finally, the empowered acceptance of this engendering deed—faith— totally transforms the human person. It creates new operative vitalities that constitute the very possibility and the heart of the Christian moral life.

I mention and stress these points because there has been and still is a tendency to conceive of Christian ethics in terms of norms and principles that may be derived from Jesus' pronouncements. That there are such sayings recorded in the New Testament is beyond question. But to reduce Christian ethics to such sayings is, I believe, to trivialize it. In this sense I agree completely with Sittler when he states:

> He [Jesus] did not, after the manner proper to philosophers of the good, attempt to articulate general principles which, once stated, have then only to be beaten out in corrolaries applicable to the variety of human life . . . his words and deeds belong together. Both are signs which seek to fasten our attention upon the single vitality which was the ground and purpose of his life—his God-relationship.[46]

And in and through Jesus we know what that God-relationship is: *total* self-gift. For that is what God is and we are created in his image. To miss this is to leave the realm of Christian ethics.

In what follows, I should like to cover three points: (1) an interpretive understanding of the Christian moral life; (2) the relativizing influence of the new love command; (3) a Christian view of the health care profession.

AN INTERPRETIVE UNDERSTANDING
OF THE CHRISTIAN MORAL LIFE

In the New Testament, charity holds a unique place; it is the principle of the moral life and even the substance of Christian revelation.[47] Christ says, "God is love."[48] This love manifests itself in that God loved us gratuitously,[49] while we were as yet sinners.[50] The best image of God's love is Christ himself.[51] Christ's love manifested itself in self-donation to blood,[52] out of love for sinners and to manifest his affection for the Father.[53] Life, therefore, in the eyes of Christ, consists in donation of self from love to the Father and to sinners.

The Christ-event revealed that we are destined to be one with him in the Mystical Body.[54] Clothed with Christ in baptism we must take on his ways and mature to his stature,[55] even to the point where we can say, "it is no longer I who live, but Christ lives in me."[56] The moral life, therefore, reproduces in the Christian the moral attitudes of Christ himself. This will be a following of Christ,[57] which means to love God by keeping his commandments,[58] and to love one's neighbor as Jesus loved us,[59] even to death.[60]

There is no greater commandment:[61] this love is the epitome of the entire law[62] and is a way more elevated than all charisms, a beginning of eternal life.[63] It does not suppress other precepts but is the source from which they flow[64] and is the bond of perfection.[65] This is a new law[66] since it is internal, "natural" to the new creature,[67] and so characteristic of Christians that one is to recognize them by it[68] and see in them, through this love, a continuing revelation of the unity of the Divine Persons and the presence of the Spirit of Christ.[69] From these quotes it is easy to conclude with Cerfaux: "Charity is the normal occupation of the Christian."[70]

This simple and glorious but demanding morality, where individual external acts flow from and express charity like rays of the sun, was described by Saint Paul as being "in the Lord." Saint Thomas Aquinas summarized it with a sweeping dictum: Charity is the form of the virtues.

The meaning of the Thomistic assertion will be clearer when we show how Thomas develops the thought.[71] First of all, he shows how charity is the form of all virtuous *acts*. His reasoning can be outlined as follows. That which ordains an act to its end gives it its form. But charity gives form to all virtuous acts. The form of which Thomas speaks does not destroy the individuality of acts and make them all uniquely and identically acts of charity only (a kind of "love monism"). Rather the gist of his thought is that actions possess ultimate meaning (we used to say "supernatural perfection") only insofar as they are caught up in the conferred divine life. And in the new creature it is the term *charity* that expresses this "being caught up in," this "being grasped by God in Christ," this ordering to the end, this animating or forming.

Thomas moves on to the virtues themselves, the origins of these acts, and says that charity is the form of these virtues. Charity does not destroy or replace the virtues; but the virtues are rooted in and depend on charity, and in such a way that there is no true virtue in the fullest sense without charity. Thus the virtues, while retaining their identity, are participants in charity so that they and their acts are in some sense also emanations of and acts of charity. Or, as Thomas puts it, at a single battle command from their leader, one soldier draws his sword, another prepares his horse, and so on. All are alive in their own way with this single stimulus. This is, in brief and impoverishing summary, the Thomistic turning of the new law, what Sittler constantly refers to as the God-relationship revealed to us in Christ.

One of the most stimulating modern reworkings of this analysis is that of Gerard Gilleman.[72] Human persons, Gilleman reasons, are, at their profoundest depth, a teleological drive. All that the person wills and does is a manifestation of this tending, which even at the natural level has the character of love. Since the person is in space and time, this radical tending does not obtain its object by a single leap. The person moves by halting, free steps to the goal of this tending. This tending must, therefore, exteriorize itself through moral actions. It struggles toward its goal through a variety of material combinations, choices, and situations.

It is these exteriorizations of which we are clearly and reflexly conscious; but this explicit consciousness is only a momentary fixation of a more profound total movement. If we fix our attention only on the exterior, representative, static elements of human action and ignore the profound dynamism, we fail to grasp the moral act.

In the new covenant in Jesus, in the order of grace, our *tendance foncière* (Gilleman) has been transformed and divinized by the interior grasping by God of our beings. All that was noted above about the source and origin of moral activity must be understood in a transformed context.

The transformed-divinized person must express himself or herself. Thus to meet the indefinite possibilities of choice in our complex life, the person takes on the nuances of patience, temperance, and justice—all instruments of connection with the material. These are the virtues. Charity is eminently each of these, just as the light of the sun is eminently red, violet, and so on. That is, charity is now the dynamic depth from which both the virtues and their acts emanate. Virtues and acts are partial mediations of charity because charity is the source from which they flow.

We might put it this way: because of God's gracious grasp of us in Christ, charity is now the faculty of the end. This is not an adventitious thing; it is the person finalized toward the God of Jesus Christ. The virtues that adorn the person so encountered and grasped by God will enjoy this finalization, as will all the acts that proceed from these virtues. Every virtue, every virtuous act, is a mediation of this profound and gracious dynamism.

Take justice as an example. If one must view justice as transparent of charity—as one must in the Christian view where charity is the form of the virtues—then it follows that charity must somehow enter the very definition of justice. If we define justice simply as the habit that inclines one to render to another his or her due, we have disengaged it from the subject and from that which confers its complete Christian intelligibility. We have conceptualized it with no reference to the Christian context. Gilleman argues that if we build a treatise of justice on this definition alone, we run the risk of allowing the life itself that justice regulates to slip away. Rather, Gilleman suggests that we should regard the function of justice, in the area of goods capable of being objects of possession and rights, as a realization of a normal climate wherein the Christian communion among persons can blossom and mature. Justice is the mediation of charity in this particular area.

In summary, then, if in viewing human persons and their actions we restricted ourselves to the representative content of the act or virtue, it would be as if we were viewing a dead body. It would be as if we were viewing the beautiful stained glass of the Sainte Chapelle from outside, where it appears gray and drab. The soul would be missing. The same windows burn with beauty when one sees the sun through them from the inside. Our being and actions are alive with full meaning only insofar as they are viewed "from the inside," with charity flowing.

This is, I submit, a defensible account of the Pauline phrase "in the Lord." Contemporary theologians often refer to the depth of our being and activity as a fundamental option, as the vertical depth of our horizontal activity, as the ultimate meaning of the working out of the God-relationship.

THE RELATIVIZING INFLUENCE OF THE LOVE COMMAND

No one in our time has catalogued and discussed the nature of human failure more persuasively and profoundly than William F. May.[73] May notes that our root sin is impurity of heart, a form of idolatry where

> men deny God by turning away from him toward some creaturely power, whether it is the glitter of gold, the fertility of the soil, the excitement of a career, the fascination of a woman, or the claim of a great public cause.[74]

Impurity of heart or idolatry is elevating a fragment of the world into the position of God. It is to take something out of its place and invest it with divinity. Purity of heart, therefore, is not a sexual term. "It refers primarily to single-mindedness, wholeness, integrity, or unity of heart."[75] It is what Sittler calls "righteousness," the living out of our lives under the absoluteness and ultimacy of our structural God-relationship. Jesus Christ is the primary analogue here. As May puts it:

> God made himself savingly present to men by uniting himself with a man of absolute purity of heart. He presented himself to men only through the medium of that purity of heart to which man himself is summoned.[76]

Christ said, "I am giving you a new commandment: Love one another. As I have loved you, so you too must love one another."[77] I want to concentrate on the "as I have loved you." Raymond Brown points out that this phrase emphasizes that Jesus is the source of the Christians' love for one another. In this sense it is effective; "it brings about their salvation."[78] Only secondarily does it refer to Jesus as the standard of Christian love.

I want to attend to this secondary sense, Jesus as the standard of our love.[79] In this sense I believe it can and must be said that Jesus' love was that of absolute righteousness or purity of heart. That is, it was a love shaped by the absoluteness and ultimacy of the God-relationship. The human goods that define our flourishing (life and health, mating and raising children, knowledge, friendship, enjoyment of the arts and play), while desirable and attractive in themselves, are *subordinate* to this structural God-relationship.

As May has so brilliantly pointed out, a characteristic of the redeemed but still messy human condition is to make idols, to pursue these basic goods *as ends in themselves*. This is the radical theological meaning of secularization: the loss of the context that subordinates and relativizes these basic human goods and that prevents our divinizing them. The goods are so attractive that our constant temptation (or our continuing enslavement, our bondage to the world, our constant need for liberation and deepening conversion) is to center our being on them as ultimate ends, to cling to them with our whole being.

Jesus' love for us is, of course, primarily empowerment. But it is also, in its purity and righteousness, the standard against this type of idolatry. Whatever he willed for us and did for us, he did within the primacy and ultimacy of the God-relationship. Since this relationship is our very being and destiny, his love took the form of a constant reminder of this momentous dignity to people hell-bent on their idolatries.

Jesus' love, as standard, suggests the shape of our Christian love for each other. His conduct reminds others of their true dignity, reminds them of their being and destiny, and therefore supports and protects the basic human goods *as subordinate.* In this sense I believe it is possible to say that Jesus is the norm above all of our self-perception, of what we do in a novel sense. That sense is: all that we are must be the ultimate standard against which what we do may be judged. And "being in the Lord" is what we are. That radically relativizes all human goods. Accordingly, "following Christ," "imitating Christ," means, negatively, never pursuing human goods as *final ends,* and, positively, pursuing them *as subordinate.* In this perspective, the Christian community (which the Lord described as a community of love) is a community that celebrates and shares its profoundest being and life that pursues, therefore, the basic human goods in interpersonal life *as subordinate.*

Saint Ignatius Loyola in his *Spiritual Exercises* proposes to the exercitant that he or she "desire and choose poverty with Christ poor, rather than riches; insults with Christ loaded with them, rather than honors."[80] This should not be understood as a flattening and spurning of human goods, but as a relativizing of them to a world always prone to absolutize them. Christ's suffering and cross was both a symbolic contextualizing of human goods *and* the profoundest act of love. Therefore, those who strive to follow him ("as I have loved you") are performing the profoundest act of love for the world by pursuing in interpersonal life the basic goods *within their context* and *as subordinate.* In this sense, both Christ's love for us as standard and our love for each other constitute a profound relativizing of basic human values.

This can easily be missed in the culture of Western capitalistic societies, just as it was folly to the Greeks. In such cultures people are frequently enslaved by their own self-conceptions and their conception of "the good life." To many, this term means *having things* (beautiful property, leisure, education, health, wealth, pleasures). From this follows the notion of ethics as creating the conditions that make such a life possible, especially expanding the freedom that allows the agent (a solitary, morally autonomous individual) to pursue and maximize these goals.

For the believing Christian, "the good life" does not deny these goods but radically relativizes them. They are instrumental to that which truly defines the good life—becoming what we are. We are with our whole being "in the Lord." Thus the opening prayer for the mass of the seventeenth Sunday in ordinary time reads: "God our Father and protector, without you nothing is holy, nothing has value. Guide us to everlasting life by helping us to use wisely the blessings you have given to the world." "Wise use" was specified in Jesus' love for us. It is nonidolatrous use, use within the primacy and ultimacy of the God-relationship.

Christian theological ethics—faith reflecting on itself and its behavioral implications—must talk like this. Otherwise it fails to be Christian and ultimately theological. Johannes Metz notes that "Christological knowledge is formed and handed on not primarily in the form of concepts but in accounts of following Christ."[81] The saints are its exemplars. That is why the history of Christian theological ethics is the history of the practice of following Christ, and must assume a primarily narrative form. It is also why the character of our moral agency as Christians should have its most fundamental formative ground in Christian public worship. It is above all in liturgy where we are exposed to the narratives that ought to shape our lives profoundly. In liturgy Catholic Christians make Christ present by remembering "the shape of God's engendering deed."

A CHRISTIAN VIEW OF THE HEALTH CARE PROFESSION

From the Christian point of view, the field of health care is a privileged context in which to encounter another person—and hence to encounter Christ. "The same Lord who meets, judges, heals, and forgives, in the solitary and naked aloneness of the self, plunges that self into the actuality of the world as its proper place for faithful activity in love."[82] This context is to be viewed as an apostolate, as the "Decree on the Apostolate of the Laity" of Vatican II makes clear.[83]

In the Christian understanding, the encounter of persons has a certain structure. It is the categorical moment for the faithful activity in love that describes the very being of the "new creature." It is literally our way of loving God in this context. It is the vertical in the horizontal, or, as Sittler puts it, "Love is the function of faith horizontally just as prayer is the function of faith vertically."[84] This is true of both the curing and the caring dimensions of health care. If we do not view health care in this way, we interpret and restrict its reality short of the depths of faith. The laity decree cited above, after noting that Christ made the commandment of love his own and endowed it with new meaning, states: "For he wanted to identify himself with his brethren as the object of this love when he said, 'as long as you did it for one of these, the least of my brethren, you did it for me.'"[85] But if this profound structure of the health care encounter is to be lived, "certain fundamentals must be observed. Thus attention is to be paid to the image of God in which our neighbor has been created, and also to Christ the Lord to whom is really offered whatever is given to a needy person."[86]

If the medical encounter is viewed and lived in this way, it would be both guided by and generative of the moral dispositions and perspectives implied in Christ's phrase "as I have loved you."

I am not speaking here of a psychological "immediacy" or "breakthrough." Certainly William May is correct when he notes that physicians, among others, "must often accept without false dismay the incompleteness of their contacts with those over whom they exercise authority."[87] The same is true of patients. Only a rather inflated religious romanticism would expect a direct, immediate I-Thou encounter in every human relation. I am speaking rather of the profoundest ontological structure of the encounter, fully disclosed in and by Christ, a structure we perceive only dimly (in faith), but one that ought to be the organizing shape and power of our responses. This is nothing more nor less than the encounter to which Christ enjoined his followers. This is exactly what the "Decree on the Apostolate of the Laity" meant when it urged professional people to remember that in fulfilling their secular duties of daily life, "they do not disassociate union with Christ from that life."[88] It further urged professionals to "see Christ in all men whether they be close to us or strangers."[89]

If health care personnel view their profession in this way, I believe we can reasonably predict three important results. First, there will be the growth of those dispositions that nourish, protect, and support the medical encounter as a truly human (not merely technological) one: compassion, honesty, self-denial, and generosity. Furthermore, it can be expected that such dispositions will powerfully support and help to implement the very themes I will highlight in chapter 3.

Second, we may reasonably expect that a profession deeply penetrated with persons of such faith and such dispositions will be transformed. The "Decree on the Apostolate of the Laity" states of persons of faith that "their behavior will have a penetrating impact, little by little, on the whole circle of their life and labors."[90] It regards this as the "penetrating and perfecting of the temporal sphere." I take it as indisputable that, in a time of high technology and growing impersonality in health care, this would be a truly desirable leavening influence.

In this respect, Thomas Clarke, S.J., has stated:

> The Christian deeply committed to health ministry who approaches Jesus with a view to deepening discipleship to him brings something distinctive to the relationship, a gaze and a listening ear made sensitive to certain accents by engagement in the healing experience. Similarly, the Christian comes from a contemplative deepening of discipleship back to dealing with health technology enriched by distinctive habits of perception and response.[91]

Faith creates sensitivities in the believer beyond natural capacities. It bestows sensitivity to "dimensions of possibility" not otherwise suspected.

Third, this "penetrating and perfecting of the temporal sphere" will be guided by the phrase "as I have loved you." Therefore it will be permeated with the ultimacy and absoluteness of the God-relationship, and the corresponding relativizing of other human goods. In health care delivery this can be very important.

The characteristic temptation of the ethos of the medical profession is to idolize life and the profession's ability to preserve it. The manifestation of this is the abandonment of patients when cure is no longer possible and death is imminent. For many physicians death is defeat. ("No one dies on my shift.") This can skewer and distort the ministry of health care, decontextualize its instrumentalities, technologize its value judgments, and bloat its practitioners—to say nothing of limitlessly expanding its cost.

Let me again cite the "Decree on the Apostolate of the Laity." At a key point it states that:

> only by the light of faith and by meditation on the word of God can one . . . make correct judgments about the true meaning and value of temporal things, both in themselves and in their relation to man's final goal.[92]

In the bioethical context I take this to mean that it is precisely connection with and commitment to God's deed in Christ ("as I have loved you") that is the best guarantor against absolutizing the relative. Specifically, it is corrective to the judgment that death is ultimate defeat. This is no signal for the profession to relax its vigorous pursuit of the preservation of life. It is simply an insistence that its ministry is to serve our best interests. And for the Christian, accumulation of extra minutes is not always the measure of best interests.

In a speech he composed but never gave because death intervened, the late André E. Hellegers, founder and first director of the Kennedy Institute of Ethics, noted:

> As the caring branches of medicine were gradually pushed aside by the curing ones, there seemed to be less use for the Christian virtues. I think that shortly the need for those old Christian virtues will return and once again be at a premium. Our patients will need a helping hand and not a helping knife. This is no time to dismantle the low-technology care model of medicine. . . . We must either recapture the Christian virtues of care or we shall be screaming to be induced into death to reach the "discomfort-free society."[93]

That strikes me as a vivid application of the ordering of values implied by "as I have loved you."

It is often said that health care personnel "need basic ethics." As noted, this is frequently understood as "answers to cases." Evidence of this is a recent book by Albert R. Jonsen, Mark Siegler, and William J. Winslade.[94] This book is designed to fit in the pockets of white-coated practitioners. Just reach in for the answer. I do not mean to belittle such a work. It is vitally important. But it is not all of ethics.

The theological reflections outlined above suggest that what is no less important is a spirituality for health care personnel. By *spirituality* I refer to a personal and corporate life-climate designed to foster and deepen belief in and insight into the basic structure of our lives as revealed in God's self-disclosure in Jesus, and particularly as this is encountered in the medical context. If such a spirituality is not developed, a gap will exist between personal belief and professional life.

The results of such a gap can be both personally and professionally disintegrating. I refer to the distinction and eventual opposition that can arise between the role and the person (the "true self"). Roles, of course, are essential for social structure. They delimit behavior and make it predictable. We expect physicians and nurses to act in certain ways; when they play their roles in response to societal needs there is harmony in the system.

But such roles do not necessarily reflect the true self. If one constantly relates to others through a role, one can become alienated from one's true self. The role may grow, but not the true self: that is, the qualities that nourish human exchange (patience, other-concern, communication, compassion, listening, caring) will be restricted to the role. They will become an "assumed manner," an adopted etiquette that will not hold up very long. The true self will remain anemic, infantile, and immature. At this point, health care ceases to be a personal apostolate; it becomes a job. When that happens, patients become depersonalized objects.

This is a particularly dangerous trap for health care personnel and especially for physicians because their role is so exacting and demanding. The physician must be concerned and caring, yet a certain detachment is needed to serve patients' best interests. The physician is a father or mother hearing secrets, often of abuse and spiritual malaise. At times he or she must give gentle orders. Professional expertise is mandatory. Too many mistakes cannot be tolerated. The physician must relate coordinatingly with a whole network of health care personnel, especially nurses. The physician is a government employee (Medicare, Medicaid), a consoler and comforter of the dying and their families. Many patients who consume his or her time are not sick, or not as sick as they think.

The physician is under great presssure, a pressure that can exhaust the qualities of patience, compassion, concern for others, and communication in the role, leaving the personal self stunted. A spirituality should aid enormously in preventing such a collapse.

No one can devise a spirituality adequate for everyone. The challenge upon each of us is to establish a daily climate that reveals and reinforces the contours of our Christian faith. There is not space here to enter into the particulars of this type of program (what we might call a continuing examination of consciousness). Suffice it to say that no Christian health care deliverer is exempted from the implications of Sittler's statement that "prayer is the function of faith vertically."[95]

It is reflections such as these that are suggested by the terms health and healing in the Catholic tradition, and by the general notion of well-being.

·3·

Morality

E. *From what has been said it is clear that the Catholic health institution exists to care. However, the best way to care in particular circumstances is not always perfectly clear, since values often come into conflict with one another. For help and guidance in resolving these conflicts, no source of moral knowledge should be neglected. Sources include: the experience of the health care and larger Christian communities, the local bishop, moral theologians, and Church documents. In moral questions debated by moral theologians in the Church, Catholic tradition upholds the liberty to follow opinions which seem more in conformity with standards of good health care.*

22. *As health care becomes more and more complex, there is a greater need for institution-wide deliberation on the ethical dimensions of decisions. One method of addressing this need is through committees which deal specifically with ethical and moral concerns. These committees do not relieve other individuals and groups of responsibility for ethical and moral reflection. They can, however, assist in good conscience formation by helping patients and other decisionmakers to identify values in conflict and by helping them to weigh all the elements and consequences of proposed personal and institutional decisions. These committees should represent a wide variety of backgrounds and expertise and should be educated in the processes of ethical decision-making.*

Paragraph E of the "Ethical Guidelines for Catholic Health Care Institutions" is concerned with the formation of conscience in health care delivery. It has three aspects, all of which are of critical importance: the source of moral (or conscience) problems, the direct means for forming a right conscience, and the problem of remaining uncertainty and debate about particular procedures. Guideline 22 is concerned with the place of institutional ethics committees.

THE SOURCE OF MORAL PROBLEMS

Paragraph E states that "values often come into conflict with one another." Examples of this abound in health care delivery. For example, if a physician tells the truth he or she may risk hurting a patient's psychic or physical health. But if he or she does not tell the truth, there can be both a gradual loss of truthfulness and possible harm to the profession, in addition to the reduction of patient autonomy. Here we have two duties: the duty to speak the truth and the duty to seek the patient's overall good. Behind such duties are two *values* in play: the inner need to express oneself truthfully and the need to ensure the patient's overall well-being, including self-determination in health care matters. At times the physician feels morally incapable of embodying these two values in his or her conduct.

Our concrete actions to achieve a good may sometimes bring about evil results. Medicines that seem to work miracles sometimes have noxious side effects. Life-saving surgery can leave the patient crippled and humiliated. Protecting confidentiality occasionally means deceiving others. The attempt to be beneficent may conflict with patient autonomy.

The roots of our conflicts are twofold: our sinfulness and our finitude. In Romans 7:10–21, Saint Paul said:

> For I do not do the good that I want but the evil I do not want is what I do. Now if I do what I do not want, it is no longer I that do it, but sin which dwells within me. So I find it to be a law that when I want to do right, evil lies close at hand.

This is a simple statement of the human dilemma; it has been repeated many thousands of times—in poetry, on the stage, in confessionals, on the lips of lovers seeking forgiveness, in the solitary murmur of the individual heart. The jar of our ancient fall profoundly dislocated our whole being and threw us out of harmony, and even as redeemed we must daily die if we are to live. J. Robert Oppenheimer testified to this dislocation when he reportedly stated that,

> in some sense, which no vulgarity, no humor, no overstatement can quite extinguish, the physicists have known sin, and this is a knowledge which they cannot lose.[1]

Augustine felt that "whatever we are, we are not what we ought to be." Goethe regretted that God made only one person when there was material in him for two: a rogue and a gentleman. Disraeli rendered it as follows:

"Youth is a blunder; manhood is a struggle; old age is a regret." *Simul justus et peccator* is but a lapidary identification of one aspect of the human condition. We have been redeemed, yes; but we need daily redemption. We must grow into the fullness of our redemption.

Human creaturehood and finitude is another aspect of the human condition. Human beings are not disincarnated spirits with instantaneous understanding and freedom. Their knowledge comes slowly, painfully, processively. Their freedom is a gradual achievement. Their choices are limited by space, time, and matter. The good they achieve is often at the expense of the good left undone or the evil caused. In Bergson's words, "Every choice is a sacrifice." Every commission involves an omission. Thus our choices are mixed, ambiguous. This intertwining of good and evil in our choices brings ambiguity into the world. The limitations of human beings become eventually the limitations of the world, and the limitations of the world return to us in the form of tragic conflict situations. Thus the good we do is rarely untainted by hurt, deprivation, imperfection. Our ethical acts are, at best, faint approximations of the kingdom that is to come. We must kill to preserve life and freedom; we protect one through the pain of another; our education must at times be punitive; our health is preserved at times by pain and disfiguring mutilation; we protect our secrets by misstatements and our marriages and population by contraception and sterilization.

Christian theologians have struggled with these conflicts for centuries in an effort to contain and reduce them, but above all to discover whether, when, and by what criteria it remains Christian to pursue the good at the cost of evil, or more technically, to discern the rightfulness and wrongfulness of our conduct, especially in situations of conflict.

Paragraph E does not enter into the lively contemporary Catholic debates about the method of solving such conflicts. It contents itself with indicating some of the sources for conflict resolution.

THE MEANS FOR FORMING A CORRECT CONSCIENCE

Paragraph E refers to several sources that provide "help and guidance." That wording is instructive. The sources mentioned *enlighten* conscience; they do not *replace* it. There are applications of the well-formed conscience that cannot be preprogrammed. They remain the individual's responsibility. This is so because of the individual, complex, and changing character of the choices that must be discerned by the well-formed conscience. In this sense we must distinguish carefully between rules to apply (which *make* a decision) and principles to follow (which *structure* a decision). The Guidelines discussed here pertain to the latter.

Furthermore, the very idea of conscience "helped and guided" by sources outside the individual may strike some people as quaint and naively paternalistic. But not so for the Catholic, especially one familiar with tradition. For the Catholic, the primacy of conscience has never meant an isolated individualism in conscience formation. It does not suggest that we abandon consultation in the formation of conscience. It does not say that we decide by ourselves what is right and wrong. We are members of a community and we form our consciences in a community, a community of experience, memory, and reflection. People who think themselves autonomous in the formation of conscience are roughly analogous to patients who make their own diagnoses. Theirs is a path to the intensive care unit, and eventually to the morgue. It can be no less so in the moral-spiritual life.

Paragraph E states that "no source of moral knowledge should be neglected." This may seem obvious. After all, if we are looking for moral knowledge, then clearly any source that provides it must be consulted; otherwise our search is either incompetent or insincere. But the matter is not that simple. The statement is meant to reflect and correct a historical imbalance that has developed over the decades. This imbalance can be traced to the increasing centralization of authority in the Church from the last quarter of the nineteenth century to the Second Vatican Council. During that period, the teaching function in the Church became so identified with official papal formulations that other sources of moral knowledge were neglected. Yves Congar, O.P., notes that the encyclical *Humani generis* brought these developments to a high point in two ways:

> (1) The ordinary magisterium of the pope demands a total obedience— "he who hears you hears me." (2) The (or one) role of theologians is to justify the pronouncements of the magisterium.[2]

Much has changed in the past twenty years. But before discussing these recent developments, it is necessary to advert to the fact that among the sources for conscience formation on health care delivery problems Sacred Scripture is not mentioned. Was this a terrible oversight?

No. We must remember that we are dealing with some very *concrete* and *contemporary* problems. In facing health care delivery problems there are at least three attitudes toward the influences of Scripture (and faith sources more generally) on them: first, Scripture has nothing to say to such problems; second, Scripture provides concrete answers to such problems;

and third, neither the first nor the second, but the sources of faith do enlighten such problems.

The first attitude represents a kind of neorationalism that would reduce the dimensions of human experience and human problems to those discoverable by rational insight and analysis. That would be to collapse the mystery that is the human person and the world. The second attitude is a form of medical-moral fundamentalism that would use Scripture as a kind of "truth cabinet," finding answers there to questions about which the sacred writers were totally ignorant.

The third perspective has corresponded more closely to the Catholic idea. Vatican II put it as follows:

> Faith throws a new light on everything, manifests God's design for man's total vocation, and thus directs the mind to solutions which are fully human.[3]

It further stated:

> But only God who created man to His own image and ransoms him from sin provides a fully adequate answer to these questions. This He does through what He has revealed in Christ His son, who became man. Whoever follows after Christ, the perfect man, becomes himself more a man.[4]

In dealing with concrete moral problems, the Catholic tradition has encapsulated the way faith "directs the mind to solutions" in the phrase "reason informed by faith." Thus Pius XII, when speaking of the suppression of consciousness, stated that it was "permitted by natural morality and *in keeping with* the spirit of the Gospel."[5] The Sacred Congregation for the Doctrine of the Faith in its excellent "Declaration on Euthanasia" referred to "human and Christian prudence" as if they interpenetrated each other.[6] "Reason informed by faith," therefore, is neither reason *replaced* by faith or reason *without* faith. It is reason shaped by faith, and this shaping takes the form of perspectives, themes, and insights associated with the Christian story that aid us to construe the world. For this reason Franz Böckle of the University of Bonn argues that faith and its sources have a direct influence on "morally relevant insights," not on concrete "moral judgments."[7] Scripture nourishes our overall perspectives, telling us through Christ the kinds of people we ought to be and become, and the type of world we ought to create. It does not give us concrete answers to tragic conflict cases or relieve us of the messy and arduous work of search, deliberation, and discussion.

If the Catholic approach to the problems of health and medicine is to be properly understood, we must dwell at some length on precisely how Scripture "nourishes our overall perspectives," and what form is taken by the perspectives, themes, and insights associated with the Christian story.

To see how Christian perspectives, themes, and insights are related to medical ethics, let us isolate some key elements of the Christian story and from a Catholic reading and living of it. One might not be too far off with the following list.

God is the author and preserver of life. We are "made in God's image."

Thus, life is a gift, a trust. It has great worth because of the value God is placing on it.

God places great value on it because he is also (besides being author) the end and purpose of life.

We are on a pilgrimage, having here no lasting home.

God has dealt with us in many ways. But his supreme epiphany of himself (and our potential selves) is his son, Jesus Christ.

In Jesus' life, death, and resurrection we have been totally transformed into "new creatures," into a community of the transformed. Sin and death have met their victor.

The ultimate significance of our lives consists in developing this new life.

The Spirit is given to us to guide and inspire us on this journey.

The ultimate destiny of our combined journeys is the "coming of the kingdom," the return of the glorified Christ to claim the redeemed world.

Thus, we are offered in and through Jesus Christ eternal life. Just as Jesus has overcome death (and now lives), so will we who cling to him, placing our faith and hope in him and taking him as our law and model.

This Good News, this covenant with us, has been entrusted to a people, a people to be nourished and instructed by shepherds.

This people should continuously remember, and thereby make present, Christ in his death and resurrection at the eucharistic meal.

The chief and central manifestation of this new life in Christ is love for each other (not a flaccid "niceness," but a love that shapes itself in concrete forms of justice, gratitude, forbearance, chastity, etc.).

If we are thinking *theologically* about the ethical problems of biomedicine, it is out of such a framework, context, or story that we will think. The very meaning, purpose, and value of human life is grounded and ultimately explained by this story. Since that is the case, the story itself is the overarching foundation and criterion of morality. It stands in judgment of all human meaning and actions. Actions that are incompatible with this story are thereby morally wrong. The "Declaration on Euthanasia" referred to "Christ, who through his life, death, and resurrection, has given *a new meaning to existence.*"[8] If that is true (and Christians believe it is), then to neglect that meaning is to neglect the most important thing about ourselves, to cut ourselves off from the fullness of our own reality.

The Christian story tells us the ultimate meaning of ourselves and the world. In doing so, it tells us the kind of people we ought to be, the goods we ought to pursue, the dangers we ought to avoid, the kind of world we ought to seek. It provides the backdrop or framework that ought to shape our individual decisions. When decision making is separated from this framework, it loses its perspective. It becomes a merely rationalistic and sterile ethic subject to the distortions of self-interested perspectives and cultural fads, a kind of contracted etiquette with no relation to the ultimate meaning of persons. (Indeed, even when our deliberations are nourished by the biblical narratives, they do not escape the *reliquiae peccati* in us.)

A medical symbol of this separation is a statement of Terry Kennedy, a spokesman for Nassau Hospital in the Brother Fox case. Kennedy stated: "Our mission is to do all that we can to maintain life." The implication is that mere physiological functioning has a human value as such and must be maintained. The Christian story will not, in my judgment, support this. Once a value judgment is separated from the story that displays our meaning, it begins to be controlled by technological considerations alone. This is the crux of my problem with Paul Ramsey's "medical indications policy" with regard to the dying—such judgments are never exclusively scientific in character.[9]

Here we come to the inherent danger of medicine as practiced in Western secularized society. In such a society the story that reveals the meaning of life is no longer widely functional. Meaning must be derived elsewhere, and decisions shaped in other ways. Thus in our secularized society we have the assertion of autonomy as the controlling value of the person and the canonization of pluralism as instrumental to it. The modern liberal secularized society sees its task as protecting the individual's autonomy to do his or her own thing. The function of the state is to guarantee and protect the right of noninterference.

I am not attacking autonomy. It is surely a precious value. But it is only a
condition of moral behavior, not its exhaustive definition. To view autonomy as exhaustive is to ask the state to remain neutral on our most treasured
and basic values (for example, the family). In this context Daniel Callahan
has noted that we need to develop "general solutions and binding group
norms . . . that are of more than a consensual or procedural kind."[10] He
continues:

> If personal morality comes down to nothing more than the exercise of free
> choice, with no principles available for moral judgment of the quality of
> those choices, then we will have a "moral vacuum."[11]

It is precisely the secularism of Western society that makes the humane
use of our technology seem so problematic. We have distanced ourselves
from the very matrix (story) that is the only complete indicator of the truly
human. How can we be humane without full knowledge of the human?
Considerations such as these lead to the assertion that theology is utterly essential to bioethical discussions. It does not give us concrete answers or
ready-made rules. But it does tell us who we are, where we come from,
where we are going, who we ought to be becoming. It is only with such
understandings that our concrete deliberations can remain truly humane
and promote our best interests.

What are some of the perspectives and insights that ought to inform our
reasoning in the area of biomedicine? At least as a basis for further discussion, I suggest the following six themes.

1. *Life as a basic but not an absolute good.*   The facts that we are pilgrims, that Christ has overcome death and lives, and that we will also live
with him, yields a general value judgment on the meaning and value of life
as we now live it. It can be formulated as follows: Life is a basic good but
not an absolute one. It is basic because, as the Sacred Congregation for the
Doctrine of the Faith worded it, it is the "necessary source and condition of
every human activity and of all society."[12] It is not *absolute* because there
are higher goods for which life can be sacrificed (for example, the glory of
God, the salvation of souls, or the service of one's brethren). In John 15:13
Christ says, "There is no greater love than this: to lay down one's life for
one's friends." Therefore, laying down one's life for another cannot be contrary to the faith or story or meaning of humankind. It is, in Jesus' own example, life's greatest fulfillment, even though it is the end of life as we now
know it. Negatively, we could word this value judgment as follows: Death
is an evil but not an absolute or unconditioned one.

This value judgment has immediate relevance for care for the sick and dying. It issues in a basic attitude or policy: not all means must be used to preserve life. Why? In a 1952 address to the International Congress of Anesthesiologists, Pius XII stated:

> A more strict obligation would be too burdensome for most men and would render the attainment of the higher, more important good too difficult. Life, health, all temporal activities are in fact subordinated to spiritual ends.[13]

In other words, there are higher values than life in the living of it. There are also higher values in the dying of it.

What Pius XII was saying, then, is that a moral obligation to take *all* means would be tantamount to elevating a subordinate good in a way that would prejudice a higher good, eventually making it unrecognizable as a good. Excessive concern for the temporal is at some point neglect of the eternal. An obligation to use all means to preserve life would be a devaluation of human life, since it would remove life from the context or story that is the source of its ultimate value.

Thus the Catholic tradition has moved between two extremes: medical-moral optimism or vitalism (which preserves life with all means and at any cost) and medical-moral pessimism (which actively kills when life becomes onerous or dysfunctional). Mere technological judgments could easily fall into either of these two traps.

Thus far theology. It yields a value judgment and a general policy or attitude. It provides the framework for subsequent moral reasoning. It tells us that life is a gift with a purpose and destiny. Dying represents the last or waning moments of this "new creature." At this point moral reasoning (reason informed by faith) must assume its proper responsibilities to answer questions like: What means ought to be used, what need not be? What shall we call such means? Who enjoys the prerogative and/or duty of decisionmaking? What should be done with incompetent patients in critical illness? The sources of faith do not provide direct and specific answers to these questions.

2. *Extension to nascent life.*   Paul Ramsey refers to the "shape of biblical thought" on nascent life.[14] Just as God called the world out of chaos (nothing), just as he created a people (Israel) out of next to nothing and the new Israel out of insignificant beginnings, so he calls into being each one of us. Thus Psalm 139: "Truly you have formed my inmost being; you knit me in my mother's womb." This is the thought that governs the biblical account of human life.

Of those sincere Christians who believe the Bible says nothing definitive to the abortion problem, Ramsey states that they have responded to the biblical account with "speak Lord, and thy servant will think it over."[15] Ramsey concludes that

> far more than any argument, it was surely the power of the nativity stories and their place in ritual and celebration and song that tempered the conscience of the West to its audacious effort to wipe out the practice of abortion and infanticide.

In other words, the biblical story teaches us to think of unborn children in a very special way. Albert Outler puts it as follows:

> One of Christianity's oldest traditions is sacredness of human life as an implication of the Christian conviction about God and the good life. If all persons are equally the creatures of the one God, then none of these creatures is authorized to play God toward any other. And if all persons are cherished by God, regardless of merit, we ought also to cherish each other in the same spirit. This was the ground on which the early Christians rejected the prevalent Greco-Roman codes of sexuality in which abortion and infanticide were commonplace. Christian moralists found them profoundly irreligious and proposed instead an ethic of compassion (adopted from the Jewish matrix) that proscribed abortion and encouraged "adoption."[16]

It should be noted that this does not settle the moral rightfulness or wrongfulness of any particular abortion. That is the task of moral reason when faced with desperate conflicts—but moral reason *so informed*. Or, as Ramsey says, "Perhaps that conclusively settles nothing yet, but this is how we should *look on* the question."[17] A simple pro-choice *moral* position is in conflict with the biblical story.

3. *What is to be valued in human life.* James Gustafson has stated of medical ethics that

> the most important ethical task is to develop as precisely and thoroughly as possible the qualities of well-being . . . those qualities that are valued about human physical life as the conditions *sine qua non* for other values.[18]

The Christian story can provide help here. Pius XII referred to a "higher, more important good," to "spiritual ends." What is this good, what are these ends? One answer can be given in terms of love of God and neighbor. As we have seen above, such love sums up briefly the meaning, substance, and consummation of life. In Matthew 22:40 Jesus says, "On these two commandments the whole law is based, and the prophets as well." One scarcely needs to belabor the point in the biblical accounts. Charity is the epitome of the entire law (Gal. 5:14). It is more elevated than all charisms (1 Cor. 13:13). It is the bond of perfection (Col. 3:14). It ought to be so characteristic of the Christian that they are recognized by their love.

What can easily be missed is that these two goods are not separable. Saint John notes, "If any man says I love God and hates his brother, he is a liar. For he who loves not his brother, whom he sees, how can he love God, whom he does not see?" (1 John 4:20–21). This means that our love of neighbor is in some very real sense our love of God. The good our love wants to do for God and to which God enables us, can be done only for the neighbor, as Karl Rahner has so forcefully argued.[19] It is in others that God demands to be recognized and loved. If this is true, it means that in Christian perspective, the meaning, substance, and consummation of life are found in *human relationships*.

In the Christian tradition, therefore, life is not a value to be preserved in and for itself. To maintain otherwise would be to support a form of medical vitalism that makes no human and Christian sense. Life is a value to be preserved precisely as a condition for other values, and therefore insofar as these values remain at least minimally attainable, or, as Gustafson put it, "as the condition sine qua non for other values." Since these other values cluster around and are rooted in human relationships, it seems to follow that life is a value to be preserved only insofar as it contains some potentiality for human relationships.

These general reflections constitute the shape of, the informing of, our reasoning as we deliberate about the more concrete problems of biomedicine, especially the duty to preserve life. They do not replace reasoning, but moral reasoning ought to be compatible with them.

Two examples may help, one of incompatibility, one of compatibility. Dr. Edward Kelly, surgeon in the case of Brother Fox, stated that once a respirator is employed "it should not be removed."[20] Implied in such a judgment is the absolutization of physical life that is incompatible with the Christian story.

As an example of compatibility with Christian perspectives, I would propose the living will composed by Sissela Bok. It reads as follows:

> I wish to live a full and long life, but not at all costs. If my death is near
> and cannot be avoided, and if I have lost the ability to interact with others

and have no reasonable chance of regaining this ability, or if my suffering is intense and irreversible, I do not want to have my life prolonged. I would then ask not to be subjected to surgery or resuscitation. Nor would I then wish to have life support from mechanical ventilators, intensive care services, or other life prolonging procedures, including the administration of antibiotics and blood products. I would wish, rather, to have care which gives comfort and support, which facilitates my interaction with others to the extent that this is possible, and which brings peace.[21]

Bok has identified the two conditions beyond mere circulation and ventilation that ought to be present before life makes life-sustaining claims upon us: some minimal potential for interrelating and the absence of profound and intractable pain. I believe most of us, were we to construct a living will, would come close to the formulations of Bok.

4. *Our essential sociality.*   In the Judeo-Christian story, God relates to and makes covenants with a people. Both the Old and the New Testament stories yield such abundant evidence of this that it need not be documented. As Christians, we live, move, and have our Christian being as a believing group, an *ecclesia*. Our being in Christ is a shared being. We are vines of the same branch, sheep of the same shepherd.

This fact, attested by so many biblical images, highlights two aspects of our personhood that are highly relevant to medical ethics: our essential equality (regardless of functional importance) and our radical sociality. Let me emphasize this latter aspect. It suggests that our well-being is interdependent. It cannot be conceived of or realistically pursued independently of the good of others. Sociality is part of our being and becoming. As Joseph Sittler put it, "personhood is a social state."[22]

This perspective provides the backdrop for our deliberations on procedures such as transplantation of organs and nontherapeutic experimentation. For instance, given certain conditions, I believe minimal or no risk experimentation on the incompetent (for example, fetuses and babies) can be justified. When there is little or no risk to the incompetent and great potential benefit to others that cannot be had in any other way, it is reasonable to conclude that the incompetent would not object were they capable of giving consent. Such a construction seems a "connatural" aspect of sociability. Indeed, I have argued that those who proscribe all such experimentation on the grounds that it is "offensive touching" in violation of the canons of consent often define the rights of the incompetent in an individualistic and atomistic way, without consideration of our radical sociality.[23] The Christian story does not specify conditions and protocols for human experimentation. But in describing our status in Christ as a shared status, it makes it especially intelligible to think that our well-being and the rights that protect this flourishing cannot be conceived in isolation from others.

Our radical equality before God should exercise a steadying and restraining influence as we face what are and will continue to be the biggest and most complex problems in biomedicine: the problems of distributive justice, which include the questions of the use of limited resources, of equitable national policy of health care, and of adjudication of competing interests in the medical field.

5. *The sphere of life giving and love making.* Paul Ramsey has repeatedly referred to the moral bond that exists between the procreative and communicative goods of marriage. He sees this as the nature of parenthood "in the first of it." Ramsey combines the Prologue of John with Ephesians 5 to discover the nature of marriage and parenting. As he words it:

> We procreate new beings like ourselves in the midst of our love for one another, and in this there is a trace of the original mystery by which God created the world because of his love. God created nothing apart from his love; and without divine love was not anything made that was made. Neither should there be among man and woman, whose man-woman-hood is in the image of God, any love set out of the context of responsibility for procreation or any begetting apart from or beyond the sphere of their love. There is a reflection of God's love binding himself to the world and the world to himself to be found in the claim he placed upon man and woman in their creation when he bound the nurturing of marital love and procreation together in the nature of human sexuality.[24]

Clearly Ramsey believes that we may not put radically asunder what God has joined together. In a similar vein Bishop J. Francis Stafford, auxiliary bishop of Baltimore, refers to the "ancient and momentous biblical insight of the inseparability of the procreative and unitive aspects of human sexuality."[25] This perspective of inseparability is common among Catholic theologians (Rahner and Häring, for example). Ramsey restricts this inseparability to marriage (not individual acts); Bishop Stafford would apply it to individual acts. Whatever the case (and I agree with Ramsey in his rejection of act analysis), it is clear that this perspective has significance for one's understanding of contraception, sterilization, and other reproductive technologies, including artificial insemination by the husband (AIH), artificial insemination by a donor (AID), in vitro fertilization, and surrogate motherhood.

Let us take artificial insemination as an example. Vatican II affirms (*Gaudium et spes*, 48,50) that by their very nature marriage and marital love are ordained toward the procreation and education of children, that the child is the ultimate crown of marriage. In other words, the child is the fruit of marriage and marital love. Applying this to AIH Louis Janssens writes:

> This can also be true when the child is conceived through AIH. Indeed it is still brought into being in the context of *marriage*, and owes its life to the contribution of two persons who are united in marriage. It is also the fruit of *marital love*: in marital love it is desired by the couple and during the pregnancy it is waited for in a shared, joyful anticipation.[26]

Notwithstanding the condemnation of AIH by Pius XII, it is safe to say that the procedure is now acceptable by very many theologians. The *spheres* of procreation and marital love are not put radically asunder.

Janssens is of the opinion that even AID cannot be absolutely excluded. He is the first—and only—Catholic author I know who has arrived at this conclusion. He sees AID as containing both a value and a disvalue. "The moral question is whether there is a proportionate reason (*ratio proportionata*) to make this activity responsible or balance the positive and negative aspects according to the rules of priorities."[27] Under certain conditions, Janssens believes there can be such a *ratio proportionata*.

I myself have not arrived at such a judgment. The basic analysis of Karl Rahner seems to me to remain persuasive. He writes:

> Now this personal love which is consummated sexually has within it an essential inner relation to the child, for the child is an embodiment of the abiding unity of the marriage partners which is expressed in marital union. Genetic manipulation [Rahner means AID], however, does two things: it fundamentally separates the marital union from the procreation of a new person as this permanent embodiment of the unity of married love; and it transfers procreation, isolated and torn from its human matrix, to an area outside man's sphere of intimacy. It is this sphere of intimacy which is the proper context for sexual union, which itself implies the fundamental readiness of the marriage partners to let their unity take the form of a child.[28]

This, plus a series of subordinate but supportive practical arguments, leads me to believe that there is not the *ratio proportionata* advocated by Janssens.

6. *Heterosexual, permanent marriage as normative.* Very close to the point just made is the normative character of marriage in the Christian story. In the Christian story, it is taken for granted that permanent hetero-

sexual marriage is normative. This does not mean that every such marriage is a guarantee of happiness or success. Nor does it imply that every homosexual union is destructive, unstable, or necessarily morally wrong. It means simply that monogamous marriage provides us with our best chance to humanize our sexuality and bridge the separateness and isolation of our individual selves. *Therefore* we all *ought* (because it is normative) to try to make this the context for the expression of our full sexuality. In this sense Roger Shinn refers to "a clear emphasis on the normative place of heterosexual love" in Christian theology.[29] Similarly, Ralph Weltge refers to the man and woman joined together as one flesh in faithful love as "the biblical norm."[30] This Christian norm ought to give shape to our deliberations about biomedicine's proper ministry to teenagers and to homosexuals, as well as the issue of transsexual surgery.

Thus far I have been discussing Christian perspectives that give shape to our ethical deliberations in biomedicine. I have mentioned six: life as a basic but not an absolute value; the extension of this evaluation to nascent life; the potential for human relationships as an aspect of physical life to be valued; the radical sociality of the human person; the inseparability of the unitive and procreative goods; permanent heterosexual union as normative. There are probably many more such themes woven into the Christian story, but the ones that I have listed are especially relevant to our being pilgrims created in the image and likeness of God.

The question naturally arises about those who do not share in the Christian story, those who may have a different story. If the theological contribution to medical ethics must be derived from a particular story, is not that contribution inherently isolating? Those who do not agree with the themes I have disengaged from the story need only say: "Sorry, I do not share your story." There the conversation stops. Public policy discussion is paralyzed by the irreconcilable stand-off of conflicting stories and world views. And public policy is increasingly the area in which the ethical problems of biomedicine will be discussed and resolved, a point sharply made by Daniel Callahan.[31]

That would be a serious, perhaps insuperable, problem if the themes I have disengaged from the Christian story were incomprehensible apart from the story. But in the Catholic reading of the Christian story this is not the case. The themes I have lifted out are thought to be inherently intelligible and commendable—difficult as it might be practically for a sinful people to maintain a sure grasp on these perspectives without the nourishing support of the story. Thus, for example, the Christian story is not the only cognitive source for the ideas of the radical sociability of persons and the immorality of infanticide and abortion, etc., even though historically these insights may be strongly attached to the story. In this epistemological sense, these insights are not specific to Christians. They can be and are shared by others.

Roger Shinn comes very close to what I am attempting to formulate when he notes that the ethical awareness given to Christians in Christ "meets some similar intimations or signs of confirmation in wider human experience."[32] Christians believe, as Shinn notes, that the Logos made flesh in Christ is the same Logos through which the world was created. He concludes:

> They [Christians] do not expect the Christian faith and insight to be confirmed by unanimous agreement of all people, even all decent and idealistic people. But they do expect the fundamental Christian motifs to have some persuasiveness in general experience.[33]

Since Christian insights can be shared by others, I would call them confirmatory rather than originating. I have suggested elsewhere (on abortion) that "these evaluations can be and have been shared by others than Christians, of course. But Christians have particular warrants for resisting any cultural callousing of them."[34] "Particular warrants" might be the most accurate and acceptable way of specifying the meaning of "reason informed by faith." If it is, it makes it possible for the Christian to share fully in discussions in the public forum without annexing non-Christians into a story not their own.

For many years there has been discussion framed in terms of how Athens relates to Jerusalem. Jerusalem, it is argued, tells stories but has no theology properly so called. Athens analyzes and rationalizes, without need of a story or in lofty independence of all particular stories. Thus, and in stark contrast, if you belong to Jerusalem you have no need of reason. If you are of Athens you have no need of a story.

The Catholic Christian tradition, as I understand it, refuses to accept the desperate exclusivity of these alternatives. The Catholic tradition reasons about its story. In the process it hopes to and claims to disclose surprising and delightful insights about the human condition as such. These insights are not, therefore, eccentric refractions limited in application to a particular historical community. For instance, the sacredness of nascent life is not an insight that applies only to Catholic babies, as if it were wrong to abort Catholic babies but perfectly all right to do so with Muslim, Protestant, or Jewish babies. Quite the contrary. Reasoning about the Christian story makes a bolder claim. It claims to reveal the deeper dimensions of the universally human. Since Christian ethics is the objectification in Jesus Christ of every person's experience of subjectivity, "it does not and cannot add to human ethical self-understanding as such any material content that is, in principle 'strange' or 'foreign' to man as he exists and experiences himself in this world."[35] However, a person within the Christian community has access to a privileged articulation, in objective form, of this experience of subjectivity. Precisely because the resources of Scripture, dogma, and Christian life (the "storied community") are the fullest available objectifications of the common human experience, "the articulation of man's image of his moral good that is possible within historical Christian communities remains privileged in its access to enlarged perspectives on man."[36]

That is a bold claim, and even an arrogant one unless it is clearly remembered that Christian communities have, more frequently than it is comforting to recall, botched the job. But it is a claim entertained neither by Jerusalem nor by Athens—but one that offers hope of overcoming the partialities of both alternatives.

Since Scripture and the sources of faith influence the *formation* of conscience, I have not mentioned them in regard to specific concrete conflicts. Their influence will be felt at another level. They shape a person's view of the world, not precisely the conscience when dealing with concrete problems.

Sources mentioned for the enlightenment of conscience include the experience of health care professionals and the larger communities, the local bishop, moral theologians, and Church documents (the magisterium in this narrow sense). These are all sources of moral knowledge but they are not *equal* sources. It is part of the Catholic idea that the Pope, and the bishops in union with the Pope, enjoy teaching prerogatives of a unique kind. They are commissioned to teach authoritatively on faith and morals in a way no other teacher in the Church can claim to do. But unless this teaching function is carefully understood and precisely qualified, both its concept and its execution can be sources of harm and disedification in the Church. And here we touch on what is surely one of the most profoundly divisive aspects within the contemporary Catholic Church—the ordinary teaching function of the Church (its sources, manner, binding force, etc.). The word "ordinary" is used to distinguish this teaching from teaching whose manner is "extraordinary," whether by conciliar or papal intervention. It is extremely rare that the Church teaches in this way. The ordinary method of teaching is often called "authoritative but noninfallible." This is the everyday method of teaching in the Catholic Church. It is such teaching that often touches on health care problems such as abortion, sterilization, life preservation, and experimentation.

What are we to make of such teaching? Can it be inaccurate? What is its binding force? May we ever dissent from it? The answers to questions like this have rocked and divided the Catholic Church since at least 1965. And obviously they touch directly on the formation of conscience and its sources.

Catholics consider this "ordinary magisterium" to be a privilege. Not only does it preserve intact the substance of the Christian message against possible distortion; it also guides its reformulation in changing times and cultures. Furthermore it aids us in the discovery of the implication for our behavior of our being in Christ. But if the teaching office of the Church is to function credibly and persuasively, if it is to be a genuine influence in the formation of conscience for Catholics, it cannot be frozen into a single historical form. It must constantly be renewed to conform to what is effective teaching at a particular point in history. It must be a concrete example of "tradition in transition."

At present there is a deep conflict of attitudes in the Church about authority, particularly teaching authority. Not only does this divide Catholics, but it turns nearly every serious moral problem into an authority problem. According to the Augustinian Gabriel Daly, the source of this problem is the perdurance of ultramontanism in the Church.

> The essence of Ultramontanism is the wish for *total* conformity with papal ideas and ideals in *all* things and not merely in those which are essential to the unity of Christian and Catholic faith. Ultramontanes seek to derive their theological, political, and even cultural ideals from the Pope and Curia of their time. . . . Ultramontanism treats the Bishop of Rome less as the bond of unity and charity in the Church than as an oracular figure to be reverenced in his person with quasi-sacramental fervor. It becomes a tyranny wherever it successfully creates an atmosphere in which open inquiry and honest dissent are arbitrarily construed as disloyalty or worse.[37]

Daly goes on to point out that ultramontanism is the "predominant form taken by fundamentalism in a Catholic context, and it trivializes theology by reducing all issues to questions of authority and obedience." Thus, after the appearance of *Humanae vitae*, "there was a damaging ambiguity about whether the substantive issue was contraception or church authority." Similar things have happened in other areas (for example, infallibility, ordination of women, divorce, and original sin). Daly concludes by noting that

> one is left with the impression that these areas are simply off limits to any Catholic theologian who cannot guarantee that his findings will support the contemporary conservative position.

How did this state of affairs come to be? How is it that some Catholics want a Church that will relieve them of their perplexities and hesitations, and will give them simple and firm answers to complex, often agonizing questions, while others are quite comfortable with doubt, hesitation, openness, and change? We must try to answer these questions if we are to understand the phrase "no source of moral knowledge should be neglected" in a contemporary Catholic context.

What has happened is that the many cultural variables that produced and sustained an earlier notion of teaching and learning in the Church have been radically altered. To illustrate this thesis I will discuss two eras in the history of the magisterium: the preconciliar era (the period from the Council of Trent up to Vatican II) and the postconciliar era (the era begun with Vatican II). It must be remembered that the term *magisterium* refers to the Church teaching as teacher. What that term means in a particular era depends on what teaching is thought to be in that era. For the Church's life is not independent of the cultural and historical factors in which it resides.

THE PRECONCILIAR MAGISTERIUM AND THE
CULTURAL VARIABLES THAT PRODUCED IT

Some of the important factors for our discussion of the magisterium are the following: the self-definition of the Church; the influence of mass media on learning processes and the formation of opinion; awareness of the complexity of contemporary religious and theological issues; the manner in which the Church exercises authority in a particular era; the educational status of clergy and laity; relations between ecclesial groups; educational theories and styles of a particular era.

First it would be helpful to indicate how these factors have operated in the past to generate a certain concept of teaching and what the results of this notion of teaching have been. Then we can examine these same factors and their influence on contemporary notions of teaching in the Church. There is always the danger of caricature in this type of broad delineation, but hopefully the cumulative validity will suffice to compensate for any individual overstatement.

The self-definition of the Church. In the preconciliar past, a rather one-sidedly juridical model of the Church prevailed. The Church was often described in the terminology of civil society. Such a description highlighted a vertical or pyramidal structure. In this structure authority as well as truth was seen as descending from the top down, from the popes and bishops to the priests, and ultimately to the laity. Indeed, the word *Church* was frequently identified with a small group in positions of authority.

The influence of mass media. Before the age of modern mass communications, access to information was slow and even restricted. Because opinions were formed with less exposure to other currents of thought, ecclesiastical directives did not always incarnate the full richness of varying traditions and were received less critically within the Church. This means that at times it was possible for them to retain a formative influence disproportionate to their inherent persuasive force.

Awareness of the complexity of issues. In the past, Catholic education was not infrequently defensive and cloistered from the major currents of secular life. Many seminaries were isolated from university life. This meant that Catholic attitudes were formed and maintained apart from the enlightenment that contemporary science could bring, and hence without a sufficiently full awareness of the complexity of the issues.

Exercise of authority in the Church. In the past, authority in the Church was highly centralized at all levels. Where teaching was concerned there was very limited consultation in the drafting of papal statements, and what there was, was often the product of a single theological emphasis. Furthermore, in the decades following the definition of papal infallibility, theologians were a bit overawed by the documents of the ordinary noninfallible magisterium. They tended to be almost exegetical in their approach to these teachings, and it was close to unthinkable (and certainly very risky) to question the formulation of such documents. These considerations justify the conclusions of Roderick Mackenzie, S.J., that "between the two Vatican councils there has been a tendency to exaggerate, or to broaden unduly, the role of the magisterium, and the Church has suffered on this account."[38]

An interesting example of the type of consultation involved in official documents is Oswald von Nell-Breuning's account of his authorship of the famous encyclical *Quadragesimo anno* (Pius XI). Wlodimir Ledochowski, then General of the Society of Jesus, was entrusted with the preparation of this commemorative encyclical. He in turn assigned the task to Nell-Breuning. "In strict secrecy . . . neither my local superior nor my provincial knew what work I had to do for the General." Nell-Breuning could consult no one and "was left wholly on my own." At the end of his absorbing article Nell-Breuning remarks:

> When I think back on it today, it seems to me that such a procedure, that allowed the whole bearing of an official document to be determined by a consultant . . . without any countercheck worth mentioning, seems frighteningly irresponsible.

He finds it distressing that "even today [1971], apparently, if the occasion arose, they would proceed in a manner similar to that for *Quadragesimo anno*." His final paragraph reads:

> Today people expect that announcements of the highest church author-
> ities—on questions in which the profane sciences also have a voice—be on
> just as high a level as that of scientific statements of the most qualified in-
> ternational bodies. This presumes that an international group of recog-
> nized specialists in the sciences participates in the elaboration and assumes
> the technical scientific responsibility for such new statements.[39]

Educational status of clergy and laity.   For centuries the clergy were the best-educated people in the world. Many cultural factors—among them the broad, nonspecialized character of education—explained this phenomenon.

Relations between ecclesial groups.   In the preconciliar era the apologetic, or defensive, attitude was taken for granted. Our basic attitudes were simply unecumenical. Viewing other ecclesial groups as in some sense "the adversary," we would hardly turn to these groups for Christian or theological enlightenment. They were not regarded as reliable sources of religious knowledge.

Educational theories and styles of a particular era.   For the past several hundred years, the "master" concept of education was (and still is, in some places) dominant. According to this concept, education is basically the handing down of the wisdom, experience, and research of the professor to a rather passive and nonparticipative audience of students.

It could be argued that the cumulative effect of influences such as these was the formation of a notion of teaching in the Church that manifested three characteristics: (1) it unduly distinguished and separated the *docens* and *discens* functions, with a consequent emphasis on the right to teach, and with little being said about the duty of the teacher to learn; (2) it unduly identified the teaching function in the Church with a single group in the Church (the hierarchy); (3) it unduly isolated the judgmental aspect of the teaching function. Such a general notion of teaching in the Church narrowed the meaning of the magisterium, which came to be synonymous with the hierarchical issuing of authoritative judgments.

Obviously this notion of teaching influenced both the theology of the magisterium and the style of its exercise. First of all, the theology of the magisterium laid heavy stress on the authority of the teacher and a correspondingly lighter stress on objective evidence and the processes whereby it is gathered. In this perspective Christian unity was too easily identified with theological uniformity. Second and correlatively, a theology of response to authoritative teaching developed that emphasized obedience. Third, theologians tended to be viewed as agents of the hierarchy whose major, and perhaps even sole, task was to mediate and apply authoritative teaching. Their creative efforts—their more proper educational and theological tasks—were viewed with distrust. The result of this, of course, was a polarization between theologians and hierarchy, and a growing lack of exchange and communication.

The most dramatic incident of Vatican II occurred on November 8, 1963. Cardinal Frings, of Cologne, rose to confront Cardinal Ottaviani, head of the Holy Office. He stated:

> We must not confuse administrative roles with legislative ones. This goes for the Holy Office, whose methods and behavior do not conform to the modern era and are a source of scandal to the world.[40]

These ringing words stood then, and still stand, as a not so gentle reminder that teaching in the Church cannot be identified with the issuing of decrees by those in authority. It is this understanding of the magisterium that has been correctly characterized as ultramontane. Yet this understanding is still held by many in the Church. In its strongest form it regards authoritative teaching as the *ultimate and only* source of moral knowledge and tends to downplay other sources or so subordinate them that they are virtually meaningless. Thus, in the "Ethical and Religious Directives for Catholic Health Facilities," issued by the National Conference of Catholic Bishops in 1971, we read:

> The moral evaluation of new scientific developments and legitimately debated questions must be finally submitted to the teaching authority of the Church in the person of the local bishop.

This is asking too much of a local bishop. It expands the bishop's legitimate teaching role into that of an all-purpose answer-giver and arbiter even of disputed questions. That brings the teaching role itself into disrepute. More importantly, it reflects a point of view toward moral teaching that the perspectives of Vatican II will not sustain, as Bernard Häring has shown.[41]

THE POSTCONCILIAR MAGISTERIUM AND SOME VARIABLES THAT PRODUCED IT

Let us now focus our attention on the seven aforementioned factors as they affect the notion of teaching in the postconciliar Church.

The self-definition of the Church. Vatican II provided a new self-definition of the Church as the people of God, a *communio*. In this concentric rather than pyramidal model of the Church, it is the people of God who are the repository of Christian revelation and wisdom. As Leon Cardinal Suénens has pointed out:

> The Church, seen from the starting point of baptism rather than that of the hierarchy, thus appeared from the first as a sacramental and mystical reality first and foremost, rather than—which it also is—a juridical society. It rested on its base, the People of God, rather than on its summit, the hierarchy. The pyramid of the old manuals was reversed.[42]

Obviously such a model suggests, among other things, the need of broad communication if the wisdom resident in the Church is to be gathered, formulated, and reflected to the world.

The influence of mass media. There is rapid communication of information and thought in a world dominated by television. Furthermore, the wide circulation of the weekly news magazines and their continuing fascination with religious news has brought technical theology into the marketplace. The scholar is in our time a popularizer, whether he likes it or not. This means that the Catholic community is better informed theologically than ever.

Awareness of the complexity of issues. In general, Catholics participate more fully than before in the social and intellectual world around them. This means exposure to many modes of thought and to the enrichment they bring. Seminaries have drawn closer to the intellectual life of the university. This type of fuller involvement in the secular world has already produced an atmosphere that highlights the depth and complexity of contemporary theological problems, the many competences necessary for their adequate analysis, and the necessarily tentative character of some earlier formulations.

Exercise of authority in the Church. With its teaching on the nature of the Church and on the collegiality of bishops, Vatican II began a process of decentralization of authority in the Church. Add to this the fact that the postconciliar Church lives in a secular world whose institutions are increasingly sensitive to the values of participatory democracy and it is easy to agree with the French bishops when they state:

> We have reached a point of no return. From now on the exercise of authority demands dialogue and a certain measure of responsibility for everyone. The authority needed for the life of any society can only be strengthened as a result.[43]

Educational status of clergy and laity. Educational specialization and the widespread availability of higher education mean that the clergy is no longer the best-educated group in the Church. Many laypersons enjoy special expertise, are capable of relating this expertise to doctrinal issues, and can often express themselves articulately in religious and theological matters. Vatican II explicitly recognized this competence when it stated:

> Laypersons should also know that it is generally the function of their well-formed Christian conscience to see that the divine law is inscribed in the life of the earthly city. . . . Let the laypersons not imagine that their pastors are always such experts that to every problem which arises, however complicated, they can readily provide a concrete solution, or even that such is their mission. Rather, enlightened by Christian wisdom and giving close attention to the teaching authority of the Church, let laypersons take on their own distinctive role.[44]

This is downright revolutionary when compared with the preconciliar notion of the function of official teachers. It is a final farewell to the one-sided dependency on the hierarchy in the formation of conscience.

Relations between ecclesical groups. We live in an ecumenical age. We experience a new willingness of the Church to seek answers from and in association with other non-Catholic ecclesial groups. As Vatican II noted:

> In fidelity to conscience, Christians are joined with the rest of human beings in the search for truth and for the genuine solution to the numerous problems which arise in the life of individuals and from social relationships.[45]

Educational theories and styles of a particular era. Contemporary education is much more aware of the need to stimulate the student to self-involvement, creativity, and experimentation. Discussions, seminars, and interdisciplinary dialogues are the ways of modern education.

The cumulative effect of these influences has been a renewed notion of teaching in the Church. In contrast to the characteristics associated with an earlier notion of teaching, this renewed approach sees the learning process as an essential part of the teaching process and it regards teaching as a multidimensional function, only a single aspect of which is the judgmental. Therefore the teaching function in the renewed approach involves the charisms of many persons, not just that of the hierarchy. The term *magisterium* increasingly suggests above all a multidimensional function in which all of us have varying responsibilities.

The repercussions of this notion of teaching in the Church are beginning to appear in both the theology of the magisterium and the suggested style of its exercise. First of all, without negating the authoritative character of papal or collegial-episcopal pronouncements, contemporary theology devotes more attention to evidence and sound analysis in assessing the ultimate meaning and value of such teachings. In other words, teaching must persuade, not only command. Second, a new theology of response to authoritative noninfallible teaching emphasizes as the appropriate response to authentic teaching a docile personal assimilation and appropriation rather than an unquestioning assent. Finally, the creative reflection of theologians and the prophetic charisms of all Christians are seen as utterly essential if the hierarchy is to express the faith in our times in a meaningful, contemporary, and persuasive way. Polarization between theologians and bishops is, from this point of view, simply disastrous.

We have said that recent thought views the teaching function in the Church as a multidimensional process. Among these dimensions are: the search for new understanding by asking fresh questions, testing old formulations, and articulating new hypotheses; the discovery of the action of the Spirit in the Church by eliciting insights from various disciplines, encouraging communication and dialogue among Christians, and supporting individual charisms; the identification of dimensions of the Christian faith in our times by bringing the wisdom, reflection, and experience of our entire Church to authoritative expression, either infallibly or in guidelines less than infallible; the publication and circulation of this expression in an effective way through various communications media. These dimensions together constitute the teaching function of the Church in its task of preserving and deepening the faith committed to it.

If these processes all pertain to the teaching function of the Church, it is clear that all of us have a responsibility within the magisterium (in this larger sense). When these functions are related to individual persons in the Church, it might be possible to say that the magisterium is composed of three distinguishable components: the prophetic charism (very broadly understood as previously noted, so as to include many competences); the doctrinal-pastoral charism of the hierarchy; and the scientific charism of the theologian. It is the interplay of these charisms that constitutes the full teaching function of the Church, and I would suggest that it is the proper and harmonious interplay of these functions that yields a healthy, vigorous, and effective magisterium.

It is in light of an analysis such as this that paragraph E insists on including among the sources of moral knowledge "the experience of the health care and larger Christian communities, the local bishop, moral theologians, and Church documents." If the authoritative teachers in the Church overlook or minimize these sources, then the presumption of truth enjoyed by authoritative teaching is undermined and the search for truth becomes subordinate to the instruments of the search (office and authority).

Bernard Cooke has made this point very effectively.[46] He argues that the Church needs structures that allow bishops' collegial witness to apostolic tradition to interact openly with the reflection and research of scholars, and that both bishops and scholars need to be challenged by the life experience of devoted Catholics. Why? Because, although the bishops, together with the bishop of Rome, possess and pass on the truth upon which Christianity is grounded (Jesus' death and resurrection), still "when we move beyond this core reality to which the papacy and episcopacy witness, when we move to questions about the meaning and applicability of Christ's death and resurrection, other kinds of knowledge and experience enter the picture."

In human affairs there always remains the possibility of error and the need for revision. And that raises the interesting question of a Catholic response to authoritative teaching. As noted, the preconciliar notion of a highly centralized and authoritarian teaching office led to the conclusion that *Roma locuta, causa finita* ("Rome has spoken, the matter is closed"). Indeed, Pius XII stated exactly this in *Humani generis* (1950). He insisted that when the Pope intervened on a previously disputed question, "there can no longer be any question of free discussion among theologians."[47] That was the attitude of the time and it led to the conclusion that *obedience* was the appropriate response to authoritative teaching.

Vatican II profoundly undermined this attitude. It raised anew the question of the proper response to authoritative, noninfallible moral teaching. For that response is itself an important contribution to the teaching-learning process in the Church. I suggest that the proper response is not obedience. Obedience is appropriate when orders are involved. But teaching should not be conceived in this way—and if it is, it shows that we have overjuridicized the search for truth.

Rather, the proper response is first a docility of mind and will, a cast of mind and bent of will open and eager to make the wisdom of the teacher one's own, a desire to surmount the privacy and limitation of one's own views to enjoy the wisdom of broader perspectives. It is, in brief, a desire to assimilate the teaching.

This docility translates itself into very concrete steps. It contains and manifests respect for the teacher and his office, and an openness to his teaching. It implies a readiness to reassess one's own position in light of the teaching and a reluctance to reject what is taught in view of the fact that the teaching is based on broad consultation and the reflections and insights of many in the Church. Finally, appropriate docility will encompass behavior in the public forum that fosters respect for the teacher. If one does these things, one has responded in a manner proportionate to the authority of the teacher. One has indeed brought a response one brings to no other teacher.

This "docile attempt to assimilate" is the response that was suggested by a statement attributed to the Canadian bishops after the appearance of *Humanae vitae*. They stated:

> In the presence of other [noninfallible] authoritative teaching, exercised either by the Holy Father or by the collectivity of the bishops he must listen with respect, with openness and with the firm conviction that his personal opinion, or even the opinion of a number of theologians, ranks very much below the level of such teaching. His attitude must be one of desire to assent, a respectful acceptance of truth that has upon it the seal of God's Church.[48]

More recently, Bishop B. C. Butler has turned his attention to this matter.[49] He points out that the claim of some teachings is, of course, identical with the claim of divine revelation itself. However, he continues, "to require the same adhesion for doctrines that are indeed taught by officials with authority but to which the Church has not irrevocably committed herself is to abuse authority." What is the proper response? Butler refers to the "respect that is due to the considered actions and utterances of those in positions of legitimate and official authority." More specifically:

> the mood of the devout believer will be . . . a welcoming gratitude that goes along with the keen alertness of a critical mind, and with a good will concerned to play its part both in the purification and the development of the Church's understanding of her inheritance.

I believe that is a fine statement of the point I am making. When Bishop Butler speaks of "respect" and "welcoming gratitude" combined with a "critical mind" and "good will concerned to play its part in the purification and development," he has put the matter as well as it can be put. Theologians are in the service of the Church. They serve it well neither by uncritical obedience nor by disrespectful defiance, for neither of these contributes to the "purification and development of the Church's understanding of her inheritance." If Butler's "keen alertness of a critical mind" means anything, it implies the possibility of disagreement, and precisely as part of that "good will concerned to play its part both in the purification and development. . . ." If such disagreement is experienced as a threat and treated as such, something is wrong.

In other words, the effort to articulate our faith and its behavioral implications is a dialogical and processive effort. This point was specifically highlighted by Bernard Häring in a recent essay. He noted:

> There is no doubt that for her own growth, for her abiding in the truth, and for the fruitful exercise of her pastoral magisterium, the Church needs an atmosphere of freedom to examine the enduring validity of traditional norms and the right of sincere conscience humbly to doubt about norms which, in many or even most of the cases, are not accepted by sincere Christians.[50]

This is how the "religious submission of will and mind" ought to be understood. It is not an unthinking and uncritical assent. And yet it is frequently interpreted this way, especially by those in the Church who have a very fundamentalistic outlook. They chide and even condemn theologians and others for being disobedient and disloyal, forgetting the countless errors in official teaching in the past and forgetting that Catholics would not have Vatican II's *Dignitatis humanae* ("Declaration on Religious Freedom") unless John Courtney Murray, S.J., had taken a long, painful, and dissenting course against the previous official teaching embodied in the works of Gregory XVI and Pius IX. For this reason Bishop Juan Arzube, of Los Angeles, is correct when he says:

> There must . . . be room for legitimate criticism and dissent from the ordinary teaching of the Church, given the very real possibility of the development of doctrine by way of correction and change of such teaching. To think otherwise is to sink our heads in the sand and hinder the work of the Spirit.[51]

It is broader themes such as these that are evoked by the innocuous-looking phrase, "no source of moral knowledge should be neglected." Paragraph E manifests a renewed notion of the teaching office wherein the sources of moral knowledge are understood to extend beyond the body of official Church documents, and the teaching office must take this broad range of sources into account to retain its claim on our attention.

It must be recalled here that *Lumen gentium* stated:

> In matters of faith and morals, the bishops speak in the name of Christ and the faithful are to accept this teaching and adhere to it with a religious

assent of soul. This religious submission of will and mind must be shown
in a special way to the authentic teaching authority of the Roman Pontiff,
even when he is not speaking ex cathedra. That is, it must be shown in such
a way that his supreme magisterium is acknowledged with reverence, the
judgments made by him are sincerely adhered to, according to his manifest mind and will.[52]

It is this paragraph that is used as a club against those (bishops, theologians,
and laity) who dissent from or even modify past official formulations of the
Church. Yet the Church's foremost theologian, Karl Rahner, insists that this
paragraph is an inadequate protrayal of the appropriate response to official
pronouncements. He states:

> If, for example, the statements of *Lumen gentium* (25) on this matter
> were valid without qualification, then the world-wide dissent of Catholic
> moral theologians against *Humanae vitae* would be a massive and global
> assault on the authority of the magisterium. But the fact that the
> magisterium tolerates this assault shows that the norm of *Lumen gentium*
> (and many other similar assertions of the past one hundred years) does not
> express in sufficiently nuanced form a legitimate praxis of the relation-
> ship between the magisterium and theologians.[53]

This is also the thought of André Naud. He argues that in this regard we
must move beyond *Lumen gentium*. Citing the rather common theological
rejection of Pius XII's approach in *Humani generis* (matters authoritatively
settled by the Pope are no longer a matter of free discussion among theologians) Naud continues:

> The thought of the Church has, therefore, advanced in this matter. It must
> still advance. In my view, we should not repeat the text of *Lumen gentium*
> (25), even less brandish it to condemn, without clarifying its sense.[54]

THE PROBLEM OF REMAINING UNCERTAINTY AND DOUBT

Paragraph E closes with a very important restatement of a principle
familiar to Catholics for centuries. It is the principle of probabilism and
states simply that in deciding the rightfulness or wrongfulness of a concrete
action, a solidly probable opinion may be followed in practice. In health
care delivery, there are many instances of doubt about the right course to
follow. Since we may never act with a truly doubtful conscience, we must
resolve our doubts in an indirect way, that is, by appealing to a reflex principle that, while leaving the question doubtful and unanswered, does not

leave the *conscience* itself in doubt. That principle is probabilism, which asserts that a truly doubtful obligation is in practice no obligation. Without such a principle to resolve our doubts, we would be either paralyzed (by a doubtful conscience) or always bound to the safer course (a perspective condemned by the Church).

In the "Ethical and Religious Directives for Catholic Hospitals" (1955) we read:

> In questions legitimately debated by theologians, liberty is left to physicians to follow opinions which seem to them in conformity with the principles of sound medicine.

This is the principle of probabilism applied to medical practice. This sound approach is eliminated in the 1971 official directives (now in place) with the words:

> The moral evaluation of . . . legitimately debated questions must be finally submitted to the teaching authority of the Church in the person of the local bishop.

In other words, it is the bishop who *resolves* "legitimately debated questions."

Nothing in traditional Catholic theology will support this extension of episcopal authority. And for this reason paragraph E rightly asserts that

> . . . in moral questions debated by moral theologians in the Church, Catholic tradition upholds the liberty to follow opinions which seem more in conformity with standards of good health care.

Guideline 22 is concerned with ethics committees in health care institutions. It views such committees modestly, as "one method" of facing ethical dilemmas, and it suggests what such committees *cannot* do, what they *can* do, and how they should be composed.

First, an ethics committee does not relieve others of their responsibility for ethical reflection. This statement is based on two facts: that patient-management decisions are very *personal* ones, and that they have an *ethical* dimension. Therefore health care personnel are necessarily involved in ethical reflection, even if they are not aware of it. When the idea of ethics committees was suggested by San Antonio physician Karen Teel, one of the justifications for them was the fact that such committees might diffuse the heavy burden of responsibility that is experienced by the individual decision-maker. Such diffusion is not an unmitigated good since it could have the effect of relieving everyone of the sense that they are responsible for the patient.

Such committees can "assist in the formation of good conscience." Here there are any number of areas in which a committee could be of assistance. First, it could aid in the protection of patient autonomy for competent patients. Second, it could formulate policies concerning justice, social ethics, and resource allocation for the institution. Third, it could be a resource for difficult decisions touching incompetent dying patients. Finally, in Catholic health care institutions, it could aid in the formulation of policies concerning controversial procedures (for example, sterilization).

· 4 ·

Justice in Health Care

The "Ethical and Religious Directives for Catholic Health Facilities" (1971) contains not a single directive on social justice; the word *justice* does not even appear in this document. In fact, justice is not one of the explicit themes of Project X. Yet every serious student of health and medicine knows that the major moral problems in bioethics are sociopolitical in character. Daniel Callahan has summarized this matter splendidly. He argues that the allocation of resources, the development of a just health care delivery system, the adjudication of the rights and claims of different competing groups "are and will be the important moral problems of the future."[1]

A number of issues can be considered under the rubric of justice in health care. The two that seem most pressing (and controversial) are access to health care (What is our obligation to ensure equitable access to our health care system?) and allocation of resources (Are we allotting an appropriate amount of resources to health care and to the proper health services?).

Obviously these issues are closely related. Problems of access may stem in part from an undue emphasis on expensive high technology and acute care. These issues need to be examined in tandem.

National attention has been focused recently on the issue of access to health care.[2] This is understandable, given the increasing number of people who are served poorly or not at all by our present powerful and entrenched system. As many as twenty-five million Americans have no medical insurance and many millions more are inadequately insured. The most vulnerable segments of our population—children and women in female-headed households, the elderly, minorities, and the disabled—are those who suffer most as a result of our inadequate health care system. And it is they who are bearing the brunt of budget cuts to check spiraling health care costs.

75

At the same time we as a nation claim that meeting the health care needs of all our people is an important goal, the economics of health care is causing the hospital field to think of itself as a form of commerce.

It must be recalled that our health care system mirrors our society. It is easy to overlook how thoroughly Catholic health care institutions exhibit the failings of the system in general. The structures that dominate health care bear the label: "Made in the United States." Modern medical science, the assault on pathophysiology, high technology, current political patterns—these shape current health care, Catholic as well as secular. If we compare our Catholic health care institutions to institutions in Vietnam, Peru, or China, we can see that it is national characteristics, not religious character, which most powerfully dominate.

The facts that in Catholic health care institutions the vast majority of medical staff (with the wealth, power, prestige that accompany their position are white men and that the vast majority of high-level nursing personnel are white women reflect our American culture more than they reflect the fulfillment of a religious mission. The fact that we can survive as an institution only by limiting the percentage of Medicaid patients we treat—not to mention the severe limits on cost-free care—reminds us that we are fundamentally woven on the loom of the United States, with its political and societal priorities, traditions, and patterns.

Becoming institutions of Christian priority is a monumental undertaking. We are not tuning an instrument in the orchestra; we are attempting to redefine the orchestra itself and the larger societal expectations concerning orchestras and music. We are challenging the imaginations and the pocketbooks of our society. And we who struggle to do it are not from Mars or mainland China—we too bear the stamp "Made in America." But we have also been nurtured by a religious tradition that holds out a vision. Our struggle is both within ourselves and in our communities.

Guidelines 4 through 10 are a modest attempt to point to some of the social responsibilities of the contemporary Catholic health care facility. In this sense they symbolize the shift from the uniquely beneficence-oriented Hippocratic tradition to a more socially sensitive one.

4. *A health care institution relates to United States society and culture in significant ways:*
   a) *it can be seen as a microcosm of the larger society and its value priorities;*
   b) *it has strong bonds of interdependence with major dimensions of this society: legal, economic, technological, political, profes-*

*sional. In all of these societal relationships, institutions are pre-
sented with challenges regarding justice. Responses to these challenges should be shaped by the social teachings of the Church.*

Guideline 4 emphasizes something that should be obvious but is often
overlooked: health care facilities not only affect society but are affected by
it. It is a reminder that Catholicism should not simply reflect a culture, but
should challenge it.

Take, for example, the issue of justice. Daniel Maguire has noted the difference between biblical justice and the prevailing notions of justice in the
United States.[3] He lists these differences as follows:

American	*Biblical*
Avowedly impartial	Biased in favor of the poor
Abstract (blindfolded)	Earthy and sin-conscious
Reactive	Preactive
Punitive	Benevolent
Individualistic	Social
Stressing merit	Stressing need
Private property rights	Redistributive empowerment
Egalitarian (arithmetic)	Uneven (geometric)
Conservative	Revolutionizing
National	Universalist
Minimalistic	Effusive
Seeks end of litigation	Seeks *shalom*
Avowedly dispassionate	Candidly passionate
Macho-masculine	Feminine

If the health care facility is often a microcosm of the larger society, chances
are that its notions of justice will reflect the American rather than the biblical mode. This interdependence can show in important ways. *Legally*
there may be the strong inclination to drop or curtail service from a consideration of liability over patient good. *Economically* there may be the strong
inclination to drop or curtail nonprofit services. *Technologically*, Catholic
facilities may have to forgo some high technology so that all may have better
general services. *Politically* there may be a temptation to value-neutrality in
an attempt to raise funds. *Professionally*, the social teaching of the Church
firmly maintains that all persons are equal and the Church ought to toler-
ate no dominance of professional classes (for example, physicians and law-
yers); professionals are, as ministers to others, servants.

5. *The employer/employee relationship demands particular attention. A just structure in this relationship calls for fairness and mutual accountability. Only in this way will the health care institution become a model of the justice it recommends to the broader society.*

Guideline 5 stresses two aspects of the employer-employee relationship: mutual accountability and fairness. *Mutual* is used to stress the fact that administrators are also accountable, and most especially for the overall mission of the hospital. An administrator in a Catholic facility who is merely a successful financial officer has not responded adequately to his or her responsibilities.

Fairness in the relationship includes due process, staff education, and career-development opportunities. If justice is to be served, the professional environment must promote not only delivery of services but personal growth and fulfillment.

Guideline 5 proposes that care for staff should become a distinguishing factor in Catholic facilities. Three complaints are frequently registered. First is rigidity in dismissal policies: this includes a failure to distinguish inadvertent mistakes from deliberate transgressions; it also includes a failure to establish a scale of penalties proportionate to transgressions. Second, there is inconsistency in application of disciplinary policies, and sometimes open partiality. Finally, there is a need for accurate evaluation procedures.

Does a just structure demand unionization? This is a very hotly disputed question in Catholic health care circles. On the one hand, administrators are against unions, and for a variety of reasons. Some argue that unionization would compromise the "family" spirit of the facility. Others see their major responsibility as being to the patients and not to the staff. Still others note that some bargaining organizations (for example, the Washington State Nurses Association) publicly lobby for abortion. On the other hand, those favoring unionization, or at least the right to unionize, argue that Catholic social principles so clearly defend this right that it would be hypocritical to deny it to health care employees. I will make no attempt to settle this dispute with the facile stroke of an *ipse dixit*. But one thing is clear: if the employer-employee relationship lacks a just structure, the overall mission of the Catholic health facility, as well as its witness value, is compromised from the start.

6. *Independent practitioners are an important part of the health care institution's community. They are, then, accountable for the same standards of justice as are the salaried employees.*

In contemporary Catholic health care facilities, the success of the overall mission of an institution requires collaboration between salaried employees and those professionals who provide their services on a private basis (physicians, dentists, nurse practitioners, anesthetists, psychologists, and others).

Professional staff members certainly agree to abide by an institution's ethical standards when they accept staff privileges. Yet they frequently do not receive as thorough an orientation to the institution's moral values as is required of salaried employees. Since they do not necessarily identify with any single institution, there is often a diminished sense of loyalty or a lower sense of "hospital community."

Guideline 6 asserts their accountability for the standards of justice expected of salaried employees. The norms of justice governing attitudes and actions toward patients and colleagues apply equally to all persons working and practicing at an institution. For instance, since sexual harassment is intolerable among employees, it is no less so among independent practitioners. The same is true of gossip, racist behavior, disrespectful language, and so on.

7. *Concern for justice means that the health care institution will also turn outward to meet the needs of the underserved and the poor and do everything possible to influence public policy in this direction.*
8. *The health care institution should take seriously its responsibility to work for an equitable distribution of health care resources, both within the institution and in society as a whole. This includes involvement in areas of law and public policy.*

Guidelines 7 and 8 touch on one of the major bioethical problems of our time, the proper allocation of health resources, especially as this relates to the poor and underserved. Such a huge problem cannot be adequately addressed by a single institution, but the Guidelines insist that individual institutions do have responsibilities.

The very first responsibility is to be aware of the problem. Several of the popes (for example, John XXIII), the American Catholic bishops, the American Medical Association, and an accumulating bioethical literature have asserted that there is a right to health care. Of course, there are many analytic problems with this assertion, but its core or abiding truth must be applied to the poor. Catholic institutions, which exist to be living embodiments of the ideals of Jesus Christ, must rest uneasy until the poor are served. More positively, they are asked to take on more consciously the problem of the medically indigent. Just what form this takes will vary with time, place, and institutional setting. But one specific is urged: "turn outward." This suggests that institutions should find out the needs of the poor, rather than passively accepting charity cases, and should structure their own inner life to meet those needs. It is salutary to recall that millions of poor people are not categorically eligible for Medicaid. So often in the past, care of the poor was construed as direct service. This is, in our time, inadequate. There must be systematic reorientation so that the institution as a whole is geared to serving the poor. A tall order? Certainly. An impossible one? Not for those who live in hope and with courage.

The California Association of Catholic Hospitals (CACH) undertook a study on "Health Care of the Poor." In the process of this study CACH surveyed the Catholic hospitals. The results were interesting. Eight-four percent of the sponsoring congregations and 71 percent of the hospitals agreed with the following statement: "One of the primary reasons for Catholic hospitals is to provide health care services to the poor." In addition, 69 percent of the sponsoring congregations and 68 percent of the hospitals disagreed with the statement "In order to survive, we should recognize that the health industry is increasingly becoming a business endeavor with little room for charity."

Are Catholic hospitals actually doing as much as they can for the poor? The CACH survey is revealing in this regard. To the statement "Considering the environment, Catholic hospitals are doing the best they can to respond to the needs of the poor" only 29 percent of the hospitals and 31 percent of the sponsoring congregations agreed. Thirty-five percent of the hospital CEO's and 23 percent of the sponsoring congregations were not sure. Thirty-two percent of the hospitals and 46 percent of the sponsoring congregations disagreed.

The CACH report concluded with a set of recommendations. I reproduce them here as an example of a good *beginning*. I emphasize *beginning* because the drafters of the report would certainly not exceed such a modest claim.

1. Catholic hospitals should be knowledgeable about the health care needs of the poor in their community.
2. Catholic hospitals should strive to heighten the awareness of their constituencies including medical staff, hospital employees, sponsoring congregations, and communities regarding the health care needs of the poor in their area.
3. Catholic hospitals should strive to at least maintain their current care for the poor and to increase this where possible.
4. Catholic hospitals should establish and implement policies, proce-

dures and programs which provide for the care of the poor in their area. For example, such policies, programs, and procedures could include:

- Policy statements developed jointly by the sponsoring congregation and the hospital's trustees, medical staff, and management regarding health care of the poor.
- A defined budget for care for the poor.
- Implementation of a mechanism to facilitate volunteer services for the health care of the poor.
- Verification that publicly disclosed reports, for example, the California Health Facilities Commission report, accurately reflect the cost of caring for the poor.

5. Catholic hospitals should take a leadership role in developing joint projects with others (providers, health care professionals, parishes, congregations, social services, businesses) to address the health care needs of the poor.
6. CACH should undertake and support political action to resist further cuts in federal and state funding for health care services for the poor.
7. CACH should seek proposals for the development of a specific networking project that enhances health care for the poor.
8. CACH should take a leadership role in its dealings with state and local hospital associations in being advocates for health care of the poor.
9. CACH should support American Hospital Association's efforts to establish a public policy that would define essential physical and mental health services, particularly as they impact service for the poor.
10. CACH should strengthen its efforts to gather, analyze, and report information and data that monitors the effects of federal and state health program changes and funding shortfalls on the poor in California, as well as in the Catholic hospitals.
11. CACH will sponsor regional workshops to provide a forum for the discussion of concrete responses on the part of individual hospital CACH.

Whatever concrete steps an institution takes, those steps will be symbols of a changing consciousness in health care delivery—that such delivery, to be truly human and Christlike, must be more concerned with justice. Those steps will be symbols of a tradition in transition.

9. *Minority races have suffered deeply at the hands of our society. The same is often true in Catholic health care institutions, both with regard to employees and patients. Catholic institutions should play a leading and aggressive role in redressing this imbalance, especially with regard to opportunities for advancement and respect for the dignity of patients.*

The American bishops remind us, in "Brothers and Sisters to Us," that "despite apparent advances and even significant changes in the last two decades, the reality of racism remains. In large part it is only the external appearances that have changed." Catholic hospitals share in the racism of America. As individuals we come to our institutions acculturated; our personalities have developed in a society strongly shaped by racism. This does not mean that we have blatant, vicious racist hearts and behavior. Most of our personal racism is probably subtle and difficult to detect, but this does not mean it is inconsequential. Subtle racism denies justice.

A more inportant kind of racism is structural racism. The American bishops over the years have come to focus more and more on structural racism as a central moral issue. Health care is a railroad switchyard of American structures: hospitals are major workplaces; they are gatekeepers to a myriad of services; they are borrowers and investors; they own real estate; they are megacustomers; they are large and complex human organizations. All of these arteries of American life are contaminated with the historical debris of racism.

This is not only a case of the tradition laying out clear lines of development, but also of large-scale ignorance and inaction within the Catholic community. The next step of tradition's transition is not on the level of defining a concept but of converting clarity of concept into concerted action.

Guideline 9 stresses the fact that what is true of society in general is true also of Catholic health care institutions. They have unwittingly incorporated into their lifestyle certain responses that are oppressive to minorities. Four areas stand out. First, minorities have been given the low-prestige jobs. Second, the attitudes of emergency-room personnel are too frequently neglectful and even discriminatory. Third, there is too often the embarrassment of a communication problem and too little corporate effort to help non-English speakers. Finally, minorities are more likely to experience a lack of respect for patients. Such responses, oppressive to patients, are clearly at odds with the mission of a Catholic facility.

10. *A similar justice concern about the welfare of women—both patients and employees—should characterize a Catholic health care insitution. Women and men should be afforded the same respect and consideration with regard to diagnoses and treatment. Women employees should have equal opportunity for employment and career development, and their work should be fairly compensated, i.e., in accord with the principle of equal pay for work of equal value.*

Guideline 10 may at first appear trivial, a token nod to a contemporary fad. Yet it must be seen against the background of male domination, both in the Church and in organized medicine. This domination has led to inequity in the way women patients are treated.

There is a massive change going on in the Church in America. Four interesting episcopal statements are evidence of this. The first is that issued over the signature of John S. Cummins, of Oakland.[4] It notes that this decade has produced singular discernment of the place of women in the Church and that these are but the initial stages of an "obviously new and continuing development." This statement, drawn up by a committee of the priests' senate, made several concrete recommendations, for instance, that those in charge of formation and continuing education should see to it that their programs are sensitive to and supportive of women's ministerial education and that a clearinghouse for women seeking ministerial placement should be provided.

The second statement is a pastoral letter issued jointly by Victor Balke, of Crookston, and Raymond Lucker, of New Ulm.[5] The letter was written in the "hope that it will raise to a new level of awareness the issue of Christian feminism and the sin of sexism." It includes excellent and very detailed questions for an examination of conscience for members of the Church regarding attitudes and pastoral practices involving women. Rectifying sexist attitudes and practices is a matter of justice deserving "high priority."

The third document is that of Matthew Clark of Rochester.[6] Clark stated, "Women of every state of life and nation, every financial stratum, every culture and religious tradition, are asking for what is rightfully theirs." Clark notes that some women view their life in the Church as "painfully confusing." This has led them to perceive the Church as "generating and reinforcing circumstances oppressive to them." He urges diocesan agencies to make participation of women a priority. Clark acknowledges that current norms for women's ministry "are a source of suffering." But he asks all to face these questions in an "open and communal manner." Finally, Bishop Clark proposes sixteen "courses of action." For instance, he makes it a priority for the Rochester diocese to bring women into the various agencies of the diocese. Women should be on all study commissions and advisory boards. All educational programs should include the role of women in their curricula. Women's participation in liturgical functions should be encouraged "in those roles now open to them."

The fourth statement is that of Thomas J. Gumbleton, auxiliary bishop of Detroit. Speaking in 1983 to a group of one hundred priests, religious, and laypersons, Gumbleton described the Church's treatment of women as "structural injustice" and "social sin."[7] He criticized the Church's rule against having girls as servers at Mass. "I can't obey a law like that because it is unjust. I don't think any of you should obey it."

These are just four recent initiatives by American Catholic bishops. Others have preceded them.[8] What are we to make of them? It would be easy to dismiss these moves as episcopal fads. But that would be a mistake for two reasons. First, the feminist movement has been heard in these quarters and the hearers have done their homework. Second, the very practical and concrete formulations of policy show a profound moral seriousness. In summary, I believe we are witnessing change in consciousness in the Church. The very first step leading to this change is, of course, the realization of the extent and depth of sexism in the Church—in its policies, leaders, structures, symbols, and liturgy. All four statements acknowledge such sexism.

This sexism has not been absent from health care delivery. Speaking in 1980 to the Religious Leaders Consultation on the World Conference of the United Nations Decade of Women, Dr. Ann Neale mentioned some problems that crowd under the umbrella of "justice-concern for the welfare of women."[9] For instance, there is the problem of sexual stereotyping that inappropriately channels women into health care (for example, women with certain characteristics are often deemed to have mental and emotional problems, while men with the same characteristics are not so diagnosed). The evidence for this is soft and sometimes anecdotal, but the allegations are made often enough to cause concern.[10]

Then there is the inappropriate use of technology. Let the increasing use of Caesarean section be an example. Until the 1960s, Caesarean section accounted for about 2 percent of all deliveries. Today the national rate is about 17 percent, an 800 percent increase. Some of this can be explained by the growth of the science of fetology, but far from all of it. Another example is hysterectomy. Excluding biopsy, hysterectomy is the second most frequently performed surgical procedure in the United States. It is estimated that 62 percent of all American women will have had a hysterectomy by age seventy. Women are nearly twice as likely to undergo surgery as men. This reflects an attitude less hesitant to subject women to serious surgery than men.

The role of the mid-level practitioner (nurse practitioner, nurse midwife, and physician's assistant)—a role frequently filled by women—emerged in the early 1970s in response to the increasing numbers of medically indigent people in the cities and medically underserved people in the outlying rural areas. The federal reimbursement system, along with the women's movement, favorably influenced the growth of this role. Though presently flourishing as an additional means of providing health care to the poor, the mid-level practitioner remains under constant pressure and threat from individual physician providers and organizations representing them.

Furthermore, there are problems for many women of access to the health care system. Women holding low-paying or part-time jobs are often ineligible for Medicaid. Medicare for women over sixty-five requires large out-of-pocket payments. Moreover, many women are covered as dependents of their working spouse, and not in their own right. This dependent status causes loss of coverage if separation or divorce occurs. This list could be continued almost endlessly.

Guideline 10 suggests all of these problems, problems only recognized because of changing consciousness about the role of women in Church and society. Therefore, the Guideline must be seen as a concretization of a tradition in transition.

·5·

Sexuality

14. *Health care institutions are involved in aiding spouses to implement their procreative choices. In performing this service they should encourage responsible parenthood, which includes an openness to children, the appropriate limitation of conception when called for, and proper care of existing children. The moral status of some of the means to responsible procreation and limitation of children is controverted in the Church today. Health care personnel should be aware of these controversies, and health care institutions should take them into account in formulating their policies.*

In his interesting book *The Pope's Divisions: The Roman Catholic Church Today*, Peter Nichols, has a chapter entitled "The Failure with Sex." The chapter begins as follows:

> The question of women, the question of divorce, the question of polygamy, even the question of the priesthood, contains a powerful element of sex, and if there is one issue which it is fair to say that Christianity as a whole, and Catholicism in particular, has failed to handle successfully, it is sex. There is no further excuse unless there really exists a kind of urge to be gloriously wrong at any cost, like the handling of the Light Brigade.[1]

Nichols, a sympathetic outsider, goes on to criticize the 1980 Synod. Citing a cardinal from the Third World who is troubled by the problems of his own overpopulated diocese, Nichols continues:

> He nevertheless kept such views to himself during the Synod. He knows, as so many know, that the essential reason why the Vatican will not, unless forced, give way, is that the teachings on sex are a confusion which does no credit to the Church. But you cannot, of course, admit that.[2]

Nichols notes that this "confusion" combines with an "attitude of total certainty" in presenting sexual teachings.

Whether one agrees with Nichols's judgment or not, there is little doubt that it is widely shared, not only outside but inside the Church. *Humanae vitae* was the object of massive dissent when it appeared in 1968. When *Inter insigniores* appeared in 1977 (reaffirming the prohibition of the ordination of women), it was criticized for its inadequate theological arguments. In 1976, the Sacred Congregation for the Doctrine of the Faith released *Persona humana* ("Declaration on Certain Questions Concerning Sexual Ethics"). It, too, was broadly criticized. For instance, a group of French theologians comprising the Regional Organization for Theological Development (ORDET) criticized its "individualistic and legalistic character, its outdated philosophical categories, its abusive authoritarianism."[3] Roman Bleistein, S.J., associate editor of *Stimmen der Zeit*, thought that anyone concerned about the Church's authority must wonder whether its institutions are not undermining their own authority.[4] The Spanish journal *Razon y fe* attacked the static notion of nature in the document.[5] A group of Tübingen theologians argued that *Persona humana* is entirely deductive, misuses its own tradition, is morally positivistic, and does not take scientific data seriously.[6] Bernard Häring complained that the natural-law perspectives of the contemporary consultors to the Congregation are "represented as *the* constant tradition and teaching of the Church.... There speaks in the document not *the* preconciliar theology, but a very distinct preconciliar theology, the type rejected by the Council in its rejection of several preliminary drafts for *Gaudium et spes.*"[7]

What has gone wrong? Some will argue that nothing has gone wrong. The Church simply speaks a prophetic message to a thoroughly pansexualized world, one increasingly incapable of hearing its voice. We have to expect such rejection and ridicule. Others dismiss such apologies as playing the ostrich. After all, the severest criticisms of the Church's sexual teaching comes from devoted and theologically sophisticated Catholics.

The Catholic Church's attitudes toward sexuality have developed over a long period of time. To understand the contemporary situation, a brief review of such developments is necessary. I will highlight six moments in this history.[8]

SAINT AUGUSTINE

Saint Augustine juxtaposed two definitions of marriage but never was able to bring them together.

First, there is marriage founded on the biological difference of the sexes. For Augustine, the distinction between the sexes was for procreation; marriage, insofar as it is founded on this distinction, exists only for procreation. "When one asks," he states, "about the kind of help for which the female sex was added to man . . . for one who considers the question the sole reason is procreation."[9] "Procreation, therefore, of children is itself the first, the natural, and the legitimate cause of marriage."[10] Since marriage exists only for procreation, the marital act exists only for procreation. Procreation is its only acceptable motive.

Augustine accepted the consequences of this analysis. For him, to *demand* relations beyond the need of procreation was venially sinful (only venially because it did not violate fidelity). This was the order of nature. And it worked out as follows: Nutrition is for the health of the individual what the sex act is for the health of the species. Moreover, God has given us two kinds of goods: some worthy of pursuit in themselves (wisdom, health, friendship); others are means necessary for something else (eating, drinking, the sex act). Only one who conforms to this purpose is irreproachable. Thus the natural order for Augustine means conformity to the biological function of sexuality.

This analysis was confirmed for Augustine by his analysis of sexual desire and pleasure, and their relation to original sin. Sexual desire and pleasure do not obey the spirit; they absorb it. They are the result of sin. But sexual relations are not possible without desire. Therefore there must be justification or compensation for the sex act. Augustine finds this in procreation. When couples copulate to procreate, they make good use of this evil. Beyond this need, copulation is unreasonable.

Second, Augustine treats marriage as founded on the social nature of human persons. In this perspective it is a communion of spiritual friendship. This spiritual community has its own value and pertains to the essence of marriage, to the point that couples need not seek procreation. Indeed this society is more perfect the more it is exempt from carnal desire.

For Augustine, these two concepts of marriage were never united. Procreation is not the fruit of the conjugal society as such, but of the sexual act, which is an act of nature.

SAINT THOMAS

In discussing the content of natural law,[11] Saint Thomas focused on our tendencies and the goods to which they point. He found three levels of natural tendencies, and three corresponding goods: the tendency to goods corresponding to the nature man has in common *with all beings* (self-conservation); the tendency to goods relating to the nature man shares *with animals* (copulation, care of offspring); and the tendency to goods corresponding to the rational nature *proper to humans* (knowledge of truth and social life). The second level we may call the *generic* level, the third the *specific* (to humans) level. It is to be noted that Thomas has already located sexual intimacy on the *generic* level (common to animals and humans).

The content of natural law at the *generic* level is that which is proper to humans as spiritual beings. Though natural law is formally the law of reason, reason's task at the generic level is to *recognize* an established order that God has inscribed in biological reality. At the *specific* level its task is to *invent*, to discover what is appropriate to us.

What is the effect of this notion of natural law on marital morality? Thomas distinguishes between marriage as it is founded on the generic level of natural law and marriage as it is founded on the specific level. According to the former notion, the division of sexes exists for procreation. The genital organs have as their proper function procreation. Woman is a helper to man via procreation, and marriage is an institution of nature (*matrimonium officium naturae*). Thus we have Thomas's notion of sexual intercourse as an act of nature. Its demands are inscribed in our biological function.

Among such functions, some pertain to the individual (for example, eating), some to the species (for example, copulating). Just as eating is sinless when done in the order and measure required for corporal health, so sexual intercourse is sinless on the condition that it is performed in a manner required by human procreation.

On this basis Thomas referred to sins "against nature" (*contra naturam*). Clearly all sins, as repugnant to reason, are against nature in a broad sense. But violations of the generic level of natural law especially merit this title. Why? Because this level is prior and more stable. Therefore sins against it are graver than those against the *specific* level of natural law. Thus masturbation is graver than adultery and incest for it violates the *generic* level of natural law, it violates a biological given.

At the generic level, then, the sex act is an act of nature related to the order common to humans and animals. Its finality is inscribed by the Creator in its very biological function. It is procreation. It follows, of course, that in sexual relations couples must pursue procreation and limit themselves to acts necessary to it. Any practice that impedes conception is contrary to nature because it vitiates an act of nature. From this it is clear that, in Thomas's view, the order of nature has a founding ethical value because of a notion of natural law at whose heart is the biological function of the act.

But for Thomas, marriage was not only an institution of nature. It also derives from the specific natural law. We are naturally social and must live in society. Marriage is thus the expression of the social nature of persons. It imposes on spouses collaboration in all that concerns family life—friendship, mutual aid, and so on. Therefore, marriage relates to natural law at two levels: the *generic* (institution in the service of life) and the *specific* (manifestation of our social nature). On the specific level, we must elaborate the "ought" according to circumstances.

Thomas himself never made a distinction between the "primary" and the "secondary" ends of marriage. But in his notion of the two levels (generic and specific) he laid the basis for such a distinction.

FROM SAINT THOMAS TO *CASTI CONNUBII*

From the time of Thomas until the publication in 1930 of the encyclical *Casti connubii*, many subtle modifications were gradually introduced into systematic Catholic thought. For instance, at the end of the fifteenth century, it was admitted that personal motives could justify sexual relations even when they were not required for procreation. We can pick out four highlights in this slow developmental process.

Personal motives.   Thomas had argued that it was permissible for one spouse to take the intiative in sex to preserve the other from the danger of sin. This was a kind of "return of the debt," a part of fidelity. Now theologians began to ask why one could not do the same for oneself. Charity, it could be urged, begins at home. By the seventeenth century, an affirmative answer had become common.

Motive-of-pleasure controversy.   This controversy occured over a four-century period. God had obviously attached pleasure to sexual relations. It was gradually accepted that it was not opposed to the divine plan to have such pleasure as a proximate motive, provided that spouses do not positively exclude the intrinsic ends of marriage (practically, by vitiating the act) and that they respect the limits of temperance.

Mutual love as subjective motive.   By the nineteenth century this had entered the textbooks (Gury, ca. 1850). These discussions show that a new theory was evolving, one that denied that only sexual relations in view of procreation were licit. Specifically, in the Augustinian-Thomistic tradition, procreation had to be positively pursued. Now sexual intimacy is licit if procreation is not excluded.

Periodic continence.   The acceptance of periodic continence represented a new modification to the notion of an act of nature. In 1853 the bishop of Amiens asked about periodic continence. He was told by the Sacred Penitentiary (March 2, 1853) to leave such spouses in peace. They do nothing capable of preventing conception. Similarly, in 1880 the Penitentiary said confessors could prudently suggest periodic continence if it were necessary to get a couple away from that "destestable crime of onanism." In periodic continence, the notion of exclusion of procreation takes another sense: one has the intention of avoiding procreation.

Now note the moments in this development: first, couples must *positively pursue* procreation; next, sexual relations are permissible if couples *do not positively exclude* procreation and other motives are acceptable so long as the act is not vitiated; finally, sexual relations are permissible even though there is the *intent to avoid* procreation (periodic continence).

CASTI CONNUBII

In reaction to the Anglican departure from what had been a solid Christian tradition, Pius XI published the encyclical *Casti connubii* in 1930 in which he condemned artificial contraception. The encyclical confirmed past points of view and did not surpass the dualism of those views (that the sexual act is an act of nature while other relations are specifically human).

Pius XI distinguished marriage in the large sense, and marriage in the strict sense, as based on the difference of sexes. Of marriage in the first sense, he stated:

> This mutual interior formation of the partners, this earnest desire of perfecting one another, can be said in a certain very true sensé, as the Roman Catechism teaches, to be the primary cause and reason of marriage —if only marriage is taken not strictly as an institution for the proper procreation and rearing of children, but in a broader sense as a sharing, a community, a union of their whole life.[12]

Here we have the Augustinian-Thomistic analysis produced in different words (*strict* and *broad*).

Pius XI went on to assert the moral permissibility of sexual relations even beyond the needs of procreation, and even when procreation is not possible "provided always the intrinsic nature of that act is preserved, and accordingly its proper relation to the primary end." Thus Pius XI clearly distinguished *secondary* ends of marriage and intimacy (fostering of mutual love, quieting of concupiscence) from the *primary* end (procreation). This primary end meant that the act could not be contraceptively altered.

This analysis would be persuasive if 1) sex is an act of nature, 2) whose finality is determined by biological function, 3) and this function is reduced to procreativity, 4) and it can only be accomplished within the limits necessary to procreation. However: 1) if one grants that sex relations can be licit when the partners do not engage in them in view of procreation, 2) when one multiplies the personal motives capable of justifying such relations, and 3) when one grants that conception (in periodic continence) can be excluded from intention—then what has happened to the notion of an "act of nature" with a primary exclusive ordination to procreation? *Casti connubii* reproduced the notion of an act of nature elaborated by scholastic theology over the centuries without showing that the modifications introduced over the centuries had somewhat undermined this notion.

SINCE *CASTI CONNUBII*

Two themes made their way into Catholic thought after *Casti connubii*. The first is that of responsible parenthood: the idea that the appropriate measure of procreation is not governed by individual acts but by the concrete marriage situation. The ensemble of values to be preserved in marriage and the family constitutes the criteria of procreative responsibility.

The second theme is the notion of sexual intimacy as a personal act. It will be recalled that *Casti connubii* viewed love as a subjective motive (and secondary end) for sexual intimacy. Since that time theologians have seen the expression of love as an intrinsic sense of the act itself, not a superimposed motive.

VATICAN II AND BEYOND

The Second Vatican Council explicitly confirmed the themes of responsible parenthood and the personal notion of sexual relations. More specifically, it made two analytic moves that brought together the two strains that had never been successfully integrated since at least the time of Augustine.

First of all, it spoke of conjugal love and marriage and used some of the following terms: "community of love," "rooted in the conjugal covenant of irreversible personal consent," "intimate union of their persons," "mutual gift of two persons," "total fidelity . . . unbreakable oneness," "perpetual fidelity through mutual self-bestowal," "undivided affection," "structured on the model of Christ's union with the Church," "mutual and total love."[13]

Next, Vatican II turned to sexual intimacy and it had this to say:

> This love is uniquely expressed and perfected through the marital act.
> The actions within marriage by which the couple are united intimately
> and chastely are noble and worthy ones. Expressed in a manner which is
> truly human, these actions signify and promote that mutual self-giving
> by which spouses enrich each other with a joyful and thankful will.[14]

Reflection on this paragraph reveals that it is structured around two
assertions: that sexual intimacy is an expression, a sign, or a language; and
that it is an expression of a special kind of relationship. This relationship
has two qualities. First, it is *total*. The spouses are unreservedly given to
each other in a reciprocal sharing of self, an interpenetration of two lives.
Second, it is in a general sense procreative. "By their very nature, the institution of marriage itself and conjugal love are ordained for the procreation and education of children and find them their ultimate crown."[15]

Here we have explicitly the assertion that the child is the fruit of conjugal
love. That is, it comes to be by an act which of its intrinsic sense is an expression of conjugal love. Thus finally the old dualism is gone—the
dualism that viewed the child as the product of an act of nature, and conjugal love as belonging to marriage in its broader sense.

From this brief overview, it seems clear that sexual intimacy went through
three analytic stages over the centuries. First, it was viewed as an *act of
nature* (aimed at procreation). Second, there predominated the *nature of
the act* (whose physical integrity and procreative potential must be re-
spected even though other motives and intentions were sanctioned). Finally,
with the Council, it was seen as an *act of the person* (to be judged by the
overall good of the person).

Earlier the question was raised, "What went wrong?" Perhaps some
glimmer of an answer has been detectable in this brief history. Over the
centuries the Church had struggled to understand human sexuality. That
struggle had its ups and downs, its distortions and limitations, especially in
its attempts to cope with the dualism profoundly stamped on it by the Augustinian-Thomistic influence. It seemed finally to have emerged successfully from that struggle with Vatican II's reassertion of the centrality of the
person in the analysis of sexual morality.

Yet after this struggle there appeared in 1968 the encyclical *Humanae
vitae*. To many it appeared that this document reverted to an earlier Roman
theology according to which it is possible to pass a moral judgment with
regard to the "external act alone."[16] This belief is rooted in the contention
that "the intention of nature was inscribed in the organs and their func-

tions."[17] Thus throughout the encyclical we encounter references such as the following:

> For God has wisely disposed *natural laws and rhythms of fecundity.* (11)
>
> Human reason . . . perceives in the power of giving life *biological laws* which are part of the human person. (10)
>
> Hence he who reflects well must also recognize that a reciprocal act of love, which jeopardizes the responsibility to transmit life which God the Creator, according to particular laws, inserted therein . . . . (13)
>
> In reality, there are essential differences between the two cases [periodic continence, artificial contraception]; in the former, the married couple make legitimate use of a natural disposition; in the latter they impede *the development of natural processes.* (16)
>
> And such limits cannot be determined otherwise than by the respect due to the *integrity of the human organism and its functions.* (17)[18]

The encyclical provoked a hailstorm of reactions, both pro and con. In subsequent years its arguments have been subject to detailed analysis—by episcopal conferences, theologians, and the public. One idea that especially provoked controversy was the assertion that a deliberate contraceptive intervention is intrinsically morally evil (*intrinsece inhonestum* [14]). The reason adduced was the following:

> That teaching, often set forth by the magisterium, is founded upon the inseparable connection, willed by God and unable to be broken by man on his own initiative, between the two meanings of the conjugal act: the unitive meaning and the procreative meaning. Indeed, by its intimate structure, the conjugal act, while most closely uniting husband and wife, capacitates them for the generation of new lives, according to laws inscribed in the very being of man and woman.[12]

This analysis was but a single problem of the encyclical. The whole "happening" is inseparable from questions far more basic than the issue which occasioned it. Some of these issues have been stated very clearly by a group of theologians at Marquette University.

> In the areas of human understanding that are proper to human reasoning, such as natural law, what is the function of the Church as the authoritative teacher of revelation?
>
> What are the sources for the formulation of binding moral doctrine within the Christian community?

What is the precise role of the Pope as an authoritative teacher in these areas?

What is the role of the bishops, of the body of the faithful, and of the Church's theologians in formulating such moral teaching?

What qualifications may be attached to the individual Christian's assent to admittedly fallible statements of the merely authentic magisterium, especially when this involves practical judgments of grave consequence?[19]

These questions, touching as they do on the central nervous system of Catholic belief and life, explain why *Humanae vitae* provoked such profound reaction in the Catholic community. But beneath these questions is the single fact that Paul VI returned the understanding of human sexuality to a basis rooted in the "integrity of the human organism and its functions." This occurred at the very time when many thought—correctly—that Vatican II had moved beyond such an analysis and placed the *person*—not a function or organ of the person—at center stage.

For many centuries Catholic thought about sexuality had been governed and controlled by the so-called "procreative criterion." This means that genital sexual acts were assessed as morally acceptable or not based on the sole criterion of their relationship to procreativity. Thus masturbation, for whatever reason and regardless of context, was viewed as intrinsically evil. The same judgment was made of homosexual acts. Thus we read in a widely used moral manual, "Another summary rule concerning the conduct of spouses can be deduced from the aforesaid remarks: those actions are licit that aid generation; those are mortal sins in which it is positively prevented."[20] Thomas applied this notion to extramarital intercourse. While the natural marriage act is by its very nature ordained to the generation and rearing of children, this cannot be said of extramarital intercourse. Since the marriage bond between the partners who perform the act is missing, the act is still indeed ordained to generation but not ordained to the obligatory rearing (education) of children, even if the parties involved privately envisage this. Similar perspectives dominate the "Declaration on Certain Questions Concerning Sexual Ethics" (1976), and this in spite of the fact that recent theological developments had begun to accept and apply the personalistic criterion of Vatican II, which views sexual activity as a language, and the moral criterion of its usage the persons speaking that language.

The whole matter surfaced again at the 1980 Synod devoted to the family. Among the many interesting interventions at the Synod was that of Archbishop John R. Quinn. He noted that many men and women of goodwill do not accept the "intrinsic evil of each and every use of contraception."

This conviction, he noted, is shared by a majority of priests and theologians, a conviction found among "theologians and pastors whose learning, faith, discretion, and dedication to the Church are beyond doubt."[21] Quinn argued that this cannot be dismissed. He noted that the Church "has always recognized the principle and fact of doctrinal development." He insisted that "this problem is not going to be solved or reduced merely by a simple reiteration of past formulations or by ignoring the fact of dissent." These remarks were widely publicized and bluntly rejected by some prelates of a fundamentalistic caste of mind. Unfortunately, Quinn bent to this pressure and tried to negate the impact of his straightforward words. Similarly, Cardinal G. Emmett Carter reported that many theologians and Catholic couples have "moved beyond" *Humanae vitae*. He asked: Could this be the way the Holy Spirit is speaking to the whole Church? Could this be an expression of the "sense of the faithful?" Whatever the case, Carter concluded that "the magisterium must take account of this phenomenon or run the risk of speaking in a vacuum."[22]

Nothing came of all this, for in 1981 John Paul II issued *Familiaris consortio*, his long commentary-response to the Synod's deliberations.[23] He repeated Paul VI's condemnation of contraceptive interventions, but in more personalistic terms. Thus sexual intercourse is presented as a language that "expresses the total reciprocal self-giving of husband and wife." But by contraceptive intervention this language is overlaid and contradicted by another language, "that of-not giving oneself totally to the other."

The hidden supposition of this analysis is that *self*-giving is determined by the *physical* openness of the individual act. Indeed, *Familiaris consortio* explicitly refers to the "structure and finalities of the conjugal act." The burden of the discussion since *Humanae vitae* has been precisely the question of whether the *giving of self* can be tied so closely with the physical structure of the act. And this remains the discussion at the present time.

Guideline 14 attempts to summarize this discussion. It first stresses the need for responsible parenthood and states what it includes. Three things are said to constitute responsible parenthood: openness to children, appropriate limitation of conception when called for, and proper care of existing children. In the contemporary world, the world of the two-career marriage, many couples regard children as a nuisance and simply avoid them. A decision not to bear children may, of course, be perfectly justified, as Pius XII noted in 1951. He asserted that "serious motives . . . medical, eugenic, economic, and social" can exempt a couple from procreation of children, "even for the entire duration of the marriage."[24] But his thought seems to be that even such a decision ought to be rooted in and reflect an attitude of openness. In the emphasis, even overemphasis, on the *means* to responsible parenthood, the Church may have lost the battle of the *end*, namely, to nourish and support such an attitude in an antinatalist world. Guideline 14 then states: "The moral status of some of the means to responsible procreation and limitation of children is controverted in the Church today." To understand this statement, it may be helpful to examine what the controversy *is* about, what it is *not* about, and its further implications.

What the Controversy Is About

The acrimonious discussion that still divides the Church is on a fairly narrow point: whether every single contraceptive and sterilizing intervention is intrinsically (always, whatever the circumstances) morally evil. As Cardinal Basil Hume put it at the 1980 Synod, those who experience the sacrament of marriage "just cannot accept that the use of artificial means of contraception in some circumstances is *intrinsece inhonestum.*"[25]

The present controversy has moved from contraception (76 percent of American Catholic women use some form of birth control and of these 94 percent use methods condemned in official formulations) to sterilization. The offical teaching on this matter is utterly clear. Direct sterilization was condemned by Pius XII as well as in *Humanae vitae*. This was repeated in a 1975 document of the Sacred Congregation for the Doctrine of the Faith and in a letter of the same year by Joseph Bernardin communicating this to the American bishops.[26] It is explicitly stated in "Ethical and Religious Directives for Catholic Hospitals" (18, 20).

The reasoning behind this condemnation is the same as that behind the conclusions of *Humanae vitae*: "the inseparable connection willed by God and unable to be broken by man on his own initiative between the two meanings of the conjugal act: the unitive and the procreative meanings."[27]

It is this conclusion and this reasoning—and their implications—that are disputed in the Church. Typical of the responses of many theologians is that of Johannes Gründel, professor of moral theology at the University of Munich. After acknowledging the clear and explicit formulations of Church authorities, Gründel says: "If one proceeds in a fundamentalistic manner, if one relies only on the statements of Church authority, then there can be no doubt on this matter, no discussion. There is only a clear no."[28] However, he continues, we may not exclude a further development of such teachings. "Precisely in this area many contemporary moral theologians have noted that the underlying argumentation is no longer convincing." It rests ultimately on the biological-physiological integrity of sexual intimacy. But "the biological-physiological integrity of conjugal intercourse does not represent an absolute value but is in the service of total personal well-being."

Gründel then adverts to the document of the Sacred Congregation for the Doctrine of the Faith that condemns all sterilization. While admitting broad dissent against its teaching, the Congregation asserted that such dissent has no doctrinal significance to constitute a theological source. Gründel believes that this assertion questions the very nature of theology as a science, and he rejects it. "Regard for Catholic teaching means also, when the occasion arises, inclusion in the decisionmaking process of well-founded theological opinions at variance with official Church teaching." He concludes that sterilization is a "physical evil" but it does not always constitute a moral evil "if there are correspondingly serious reasons for its performance." In such conflict situations where procreation is absolutely counterindicated, "the fruitfulness of the couple has lost its function and meaning."

Certain fundamentalists within the Catholic community would regard Gründel's statements as disloyal. Whatever the case, they reveal clearly what is in controversy: the analysis, the conclusion (intrinsically evil), and, increasingly, the concept of authority that underlies such a conclusion.

What Is Not in Dispute

Certain apologists for official formulations repeatedly assert that theologians like Gründel—and they are by far the majority—"promote contraception" and by implication denigrate natural family planning. That is seriously to misplace the contemporary debate and seriously to err in the process.

Natural family planning is highly method-effective; for many people it is the method of choice. Its desirability is not in question. Contraception represents a type of intrusion, a nuisance, an interference. That is clear from the description of the "perfect contraceptive": it must be inexpensive, effective, without side effects, aesthetically acceptable, and easy to use. Lack of these qualities would spell evils of some kind. The question is, What kind?

Many contemporary Catholic thinkers would argue that artificial interventions into the physical integrity of intercourse are *disvalues* (nonmoral evils [Schüller], premoral evils [Fuchs], ontic evils [Janssens]) that ought to be avoided insofar as is compatible with other conflicting values. But they are not to be regarded in all circumstances as *moral* evils. In other words, they can be justified in terms of the overall good of the spouses, as Gründel noted. In this sense natural family planning represents what John Wright, S.J., has called an "obligatory ideal." It always makes a claim upon married people but "it may and sometimes should be set aside for reasons over which they have no control."[29] To use the unitive-procreative language of John Paul II in *Familiaris consortio*, married people regret having to separate the unitive and procreative aspects of sexual expression, but not the separation itself. When is such a separation legitimate? Wright represents the conclusions of a majority of theologians as follows: "Proportionate, objective reasons must be there for departing from the ideal, whether by choosing infertile periods or by rendering fertile periods unproductive."

Louis Janssens had earlier drawn this conclusion:

> According to *Gaudium et spes* the marriage act must be ordered to the conjugal love and to the human transmission of life, i.e., to responsible parenthood. This must be the end of marital intercourse; each conjugal act must include a proper proportion to this end. Consequently, if the marriage partners engage in sexual intercourse during the fertile period and thereby most likely will conceive new life, the marital act may not be morally justifiable when they foresee that they will not have the means to provide the proper education for the child. The rhythm method, too, can be immoral if it is used to prevent the measure of responsible parenthood. But the use of contraceptives can be morally justified if these means do not obstruct the partners in the expression of conjugal love and if they keep birth control within the limits of responsible parenthood. Marital intercourse can be called neither moral nor immoral when it is the object of a judgment which considers it without due regard for its end.[30]

Further Implications

The controversy in the Church today may seem an isolated and parochial tug-of-war on a technical point. To view it that way would be terribly short-sighted. At stake in this discussion is an entire outlook on human sexuality—and, of course, on teaching authority and its manner of exercise. These issues are contested today in secular culture as well, as new reproductive technologies, especially artificial insemination and in vitro fertilization, present us with new choices.

With regard to artificial insemination by the husband (AIH) we may recall that Pius XII condemned this on three occasions. Speaking in 1949 to the Fourth International Congress of Catholic Doctors, he referred to "procreation of a new life according to the will and plan of the Creator." AIH "must be absolutely rejected." He noted:

> The simple fact that the desired result is attained by this means does not justify the use of the means itself; nor is the desire to have a child

—perfectly lawful as that is for married persons—sufficient to prove the licitness of artificial insemination to attain this end.[31]

Because this statement was not a cut-through to analytic clarity, he returned to the subject in 1951 in his now famous address to the Italian Catholic Union of Midwives. AIH converts the home into a mere biological laboratory. He continued:

> In its natural structure the conjugal act is a personal action, a simultaneous and immediate cooperation on the part of the husband and wife which by the very nature of the agents and the propriety of the act is the expression of the mutual gift which according to Holy Scripture brings about union "in one flesh only." This is something more than the union of two seeds which may be brought about even artificially without the natural action of husband and wife.[32]

Pius XII returned again to the subject in 1956 in an address to the Second World Congress on Fertility and Sterility. After condemning contraception, he added:

> But the Church has likewise rejected the opposite attitude which would pretend to separate, in generation, the biological activity from the personal relation of the married couple. The child is the fruit of the conjugal union when that union finds full expression by bringing into play the organic functions, the associated sensible emotions, and the spiritual and disinterested love which animates it. It is within the unity of this human activity that the biological prerequisites of generation should take place.[33]

It is clear that Pius XII, following the theology of Franciscus Hürth, S.J., viewed sexual intercourse as having a natural and God-given design that joins the life-giving and love-making dimensions. Thus he excluded both contraception and AIH as depersonalizing insofar as they assault this God-given design. And he would a fortiori have to exclude in vitro fertilization with embryo transfer—not because the procedure might be dangerous to the future child or because it might represent a distortion of priorities in a world of limited resources, but basically and solely because it separates the unitive and procreative dimensions of sexual intimacy. *In principle* this would have to be the position of John Paul II; for he speaks of the inseparability of the unitive and the procreative dimensions in the same way.

Since the time of Pius XII, many theologians have argued that there are several ways to hold the unitive and procreative dimensions of sexuality together other than in the individual act. They have also asserted that the child indeed ought to be the expression of love, but that sexual intercourse is not the only or necessary source of this embodiment. Some theologians view AIH to achieve pregnancy as a disvalue, but one that can be justified in some circumstances. Hence, the quite traditional moral theologian George Lobo, S.J., has concluded: "It seems that in the present state of the question a couple eagerly desiring a child . . . would not be doing wrong by having recourse to AIH."[34] We may reword Lobo's conclusion as follows: "It seems that in the present state of the question a couple eagerly desiring a child . . . would not be doing wrong by separating the unitive and procreative dimensions to conceive via AIH." If that can be said of AIH, then under certain carefully stated conditions it can also be said of in vitro fertilization. And if such separation of unitive and procreative can be justified at the procreative end of the problem, then what becomes of the idea of inseparability at the other end of the dilemma, where couples attempt to avoid procreation?

I have noted that at stake in the discussion of birth regulation was a whole understanding of human sexuality. That means, of course, that it unavoidably touches on areas such as homosexuality, divorce, ordination of women, and celibacy of the priesthood. This is to be expected. For sexuality stamps the person profoundly and thus affects personal relationships at all levels. As the Sacred Congregation for the Doctrine of the Faith noted in 1975:

> According to contemporary scientific research, the human person is so profoundly affected by sexuality that it must be considered as one of the factors which give to each individual's life the principal traits that distinguish it.[35]

Yet in spite of this acknowledgment, the Church, at the official level, appears to many to be incapable of loosing the chains of an earlier anthropology. This is unmistakably clear in its attitude toward women. But the chains are at least being rattled. For instance, from 1980 until 1982 the American bishops' Committee on Women in Society and in the Church conferred with representatives of the Women's Ordination Conference. The goal of their dialogue was "to discover, understand, and promote the full potential of woman as person in the life of the Church."[36] In summarizing their experience of the dialogue, the representatives of the National Conference of Catholic Bishops acknowledged that sexist attitudes were pervasive among members of the Church and its leadership. They noted the discrepancy about the Church's teaching on women as applied in civil society and within the Church itself. They conceded that the notion of complimentarity in Church documents often practically implies subordination of women to men. Finally, they admitted that patriarchy had "deeply and adversely influenced the Church in its attitude toward women as reflected in its laws, theology, and ministry."

These admissions of the sin of sexism are promising beginnings. Where they will lead only time will tell. But one thing is clear: they will profoundly affect the understanding of human sexuality and the ethic built on that understanding.

This evolving understanding will also affect the Church's pastoral policies concerning homosexuality and divorce and remarriage. Let the latter be the example. For twenty years, Catholic theologians grappled with the problem of those in a second, irregular marriage. The traditional policy (it was a policy, not first and foremost a magisterial teaching) was that, in order to receive the Eucharist, such couples had either to separate or, if they could not, to live as brother and sister. Why? In a 1979 document, the Italian Episcopal Conference notes that the Eucharist signifies and realizes "the fullness of union with Jesus Christ and his Body." It continues:

> One cannot, therefore, receive worthily the sign of perfect unity with Christ and with the Church when one is in a condition of life that creates and maintains a rupture with Christ and the Church.[37]

This analysis was also used by the International Theological Commission. It argued:

> From the incompatibility of the state of the divorced-remarried with the command of the risen Lord, there follows the impossibility for these Christians of receiving in the Eucharist the sign of unity with Christ.[38]

John Paul II repeated this analysis in *Familiaris consortio:*

> They are unable to be admitted thereto [to the Eucharist] from the fact that their state and condition of life objectively contradict that union of love between Christ and the Church which is signified and effected by the Eucharist.[39]

Yet in spite of such arguments, the official policy of the Church, as stated in the "Decree on Eastern Catholic Churches" (26), is to admit to the Eucharist Eastern Orthodox Catholics. They are not in union with

Rome and are "incompletely integrated" into the Church. This major inconsistency has not escaped Catholic theologians who have, with virtual unanimity, concluded that irregularly remarried Catholics can be admitted to the Eucharist on an individual basis, given certain conditions—one of which is *not* that they abstain from sexual union.

Yet the "official" policy that they live as brother and sister continues to be urged as the only option. This policy is clearly rooted in a notion of sexuality. This led the *Association de théolgiens pour l'étude de la morale* (ATEM), which includes the vast majority of professors of moral theology in France and priests knowledgeable about marital problems, to state:

> The single thing apropos of which one can speak of a personal actual sin, according to presently admitted pastoral practice, would be the practice by the partners of sexual union. This is why it is demanded of them that they abstain from the sacraments. But we have repeatedly underlined the paradoxical character of this demand. On the one hand, what notion of marriage and sexuality underlies the position of the Church that demands of Christians that they honor all the dimensions of their union with the exception of the sexual? On the other hand, what conception of the sacraments and of sexuality leads us to the notion that the sacraments would be compatible with the exercise of all other dimensions of the conjugal union but that they would not be compatible with that of sexuality?[40]

Guideline 14 concludes by stating of the disputes on the means to responsible parenthood that "health care institutions should take them into account in formulating their policies." What does this mean? The typical response is: the statement is false because once the Pope or a Roman congregation has taken an official position, there is no longer room for legitimate questioning or doubt. But that response, besides being ecclesiologically questionable, forgets that the Church formulates its convictions through a teaching-learning process in which discussion of official formulations contributes to their ongoing purification. Or, as Bernard Häring worded it:

> Those who are doubtful whether they can accept it [*Humanae vitae*] have to study it thoroughly, have to read it with goodwill, but they also have to accept other information in the Church. They cannot dissociate the Pope from the whole of the Church.[41]

The notion of "dissociating the Pope from the whole Church" reminds me of a personal experience. In 1980 I coauthored (with bioethicist Corrine Bayley, C.S.J.) an article in *America* arguing that some sterilizations were morally defensible. A bishop friend of mine remarked to me, "I can name you at least one hundred bishops who agree with you—but none who will say so publicly." That is, of course, profoundly saddening for anyone who treasures the free flow of information in the Church. But that aside, it also points to even more sources of "that other information in the Church." Only the extreme ultramontanist would deny the relevance of "this other information" for the formation of personal conscience and institutional policy.

In other words, health care institutions should not formulate policies as if the official proscriptive formulations were certain and absolute. Or, as Cardinal Joseph Ratzinger worded it to the priests of Munich, "Therefore the criterion of *Humanae vitae*, clear as it is, is not inflexible, but is open for differentiated judgments of ethically differentiated situations."[42]

Conclusion

Guideline 14 touches on the entire area of human sexuality. Three points stand out. First, a contemporary consciousness places the person at the center of contemporary reflection. This underlines the relevance of all the sources of knowledge (the sciences, practical experience, etc.) that can enlighten us about what is promotive or destructive of persons. It means that our methodological reflection is necessarily inductive.

Second, it is inescapable that many of the problems of contemporary Catholic reflection on sexuality are aggravated by their proximity to the authority problem. There is such an investment in authority and its prerogatives that discussion of sexuality rapidly becomes discussion of authority. Even to the casual observer, this fixation will be seen to block growth in understanding, which is our main task.

Finally, the modern need in the Catholic community is a pacific, unthreatened, open understanding and restructuring of sexual ethics. Whether this will or can occur is doubtful. Even modest attempts (for example, the study *Human Sexuality*, by a committee of the Catholic Theological Society of America) are met with such panic, fear, and denunciation that scholars can only be discouraged from the attempt. But the foundations for such a reexamination are there to be mined. They cluster around the understanding of sexuality as the radical capacity for interrelatedness (ultimately intimacy) and its actuation as the language of relationship. The tradition is in transition, slow and painful as that transition might be. Guideline 14 attempts to reflect this.

·6·

Dignity, Passages, Madness, Suffering, and Dying

Webster's New Collegiate Dictionary gives as the first meaning of dignity: "the quality or state of being worthy, honored, or esteemed." In the context of health and medicine, the Catholic tradition has developed and continues to develop answers to three questions: *Why* are human beings worthy? *Who* is worthy? *How* must this worthiness be recognized in the context of health care? Because of their practical orientation, the second and third questions are specifically approached in our "Ethical Guidelines." But we cannot omit the first question if the second and third are to be adequately grasped.

In speaking of the essential equality of all persons, Vatican II stated:

> Since all men [*sic*] possess a rational soul and are created in God's likeness, since they have the same nature and origin, have been redeemed by Christ, and enjoy the same divine calling and destiny, the basic equality of all must receive increasingly greater recognition.[1]

The same qualities that indicate the basic equality of human persons also ground their dignity. Human beings have their origin in God the Creator, have been redeemed by him and are destined for him. We have heard such statements so often that they seem dead and meaningless. They seem to float above the real human scene. They seem particularly dead and meaningless when we repeatedly experience the inhumanity of persons toward each other, their cruelty and brutality, their selfishness and meanness, their sicknesses and deaths. What sense does it make to say that someone who has spent a lifetime causing pain to others is "created in God's likeness?" How do we regard as "worthy" and "dignified" a person eaten by cancer and shriveled and stinking? How do we retain any sense of redemption and resurrection for the heroin addict?

Joseph A. Califano describes a drug raid he was involved in while on commission from Governor Hugh L. Carey:

> The final bust on October 12 was curdling. We entered the brownstone at 360 West 116th Street behind a dozen police. The place was crowded with addicts, perhaps fifty of them. Up the brownstone steps, the first floor was even filthier than at the 103rd Street shooting gallery: rotting wood, torn and smashed plaster, the overpowering stench of urine, excrement and vomit everywhere, even visible in some corners and on the floor near an overflowed toilet.
>
> On the second floor, I saw the ravages of heroin as few have ever imagined them. In our room, two addicts were sitting, one to the right of the door, the other in the far left corner.
>
> "Pull up your pants legs," one of the narcotics squad members said. . . .
>
> The addict slowly pulled at his cuffs and rolled them up. His legs were eaten—there is no more accurate word—with open sores, dripping pus and encrusted with dried blood. *Why in the name of God? How?* I thought.[2]

Why, indeed, in the name of God? What sense does it make to say that people like these are images of God? Any account of our dignity must see it from within human history. And this is a history of failure, sin, corruption, infidelity. These are the things we so often see.

But Catholic tradition insists that we see human persons with the eyes of faith. And in this perspective, human history is one of creation, fall, and redemption. Not only are these phases of our history; they are dimensions of our daily human experience. As Thomas Clarke, S.J., has noted, our everyday lives are simultaneously an act of continuing creation, a struggle with evil, and a personal campaign for the victory and prospering of good.[3] That is why our experience is described in biblical literature (especially the Johannine and the Pauline) in terms of metaphors corresponding to creation, fall, and redemption: light, blindness, enlightenment; freedom, bondage, liberation; integrity, brokenness, reintegration; health, sickness, healing; peace, estrangement, reconciliation.

Our lives are processes of enlightenment, liberation, reintegration, healing, reconciliation. These words are active and transitional. They suggest the past, acknowledge the ambiguous present, but point to the glorious future. We are in the process of being redeemed. And that is our glory, our dignity, our worthiness. It is a conferred dignity, conferred by God's costly love of us in his Christ, a point already elaborated in chapter 2. Creation, fall, and redemption: these are our history as a people, and our personal spiritual constitution. God's Christ tells us what God thinks of us, and therefore we are—in spite of darkness, estrangement, sickness, and brokenness —basically lovable.

The very foundation of human dignity dictates, by immediate and easy inference, *who* is to be considered worthy: every individual, regardless of condition. But in the contemporary world, several classes of individuals are under particular threat: the sick and the dying, fetuses, defective newborns, the retarded, the aged.

THE DIGNITY OF THE SICK AND THE DYING

11. *The patient is the primary decisionmaker in all choices regarding health and treatment. This means that he or she is the first decisionmaker, the one who is presumed to make initial choices based on his or her beliefs and values. Other secondary decisionmakers also have responsibilities. When the patient is legally incompetent or otherwise unable to take the initiative, an agent for the patient—normally the next of kin unless the patient has previously designated someone else or the next of kin is disqualified—has the responsibility to try to determine what the patient would have chosen, or, if that is impossible, what is in the patient's best interest.*

    Health care professionals are also secondary decisionmakers, with responsibility to provide aid and care for the patient to the extent it is consistent with their own beliefs and values. Hospital policies and practices must recognize this set of responsibilities. Health care professionals are responsible for giving sufficient information and for providing adequate support to the patient to enable her/him to make knowledgeable decisions about appropriate care. It should be recognized that assistance in the decisionmaking process is an essential part of health care. Informed consent policies and documents should be geared to enhancing patient autonomy and protection, never primarily to protecting hospitals and health care workers from litigation.

21. *Though suffering and death are realities that cannot be eliminated, appropriate means should be taken to reduce suffering and preserve life. What means are appropriate is determined by a due proportion between the burden and the benefit of the treatment to the patient. If the treatment would only secure a precarious and burdensome prolongation of life, it may be refused by the patient or the family on behalf of the patient. Medications and other therapies whose purpose is to alleviate pain may be given as needed, with the consent of the pa-*

tient or his or her agent, even if a side effect is the shortening of life. A person who is dying presents the health care team with one of its greatest challenges and opportunities. It is the challenge and opportunity to be with the dying and the family in a way which reproduces and mediates the fullest and final sense of Christ's healing love. Any medical treatment at this critical point must aim not at simply prolonging life, but at reducing the human diminishments of the dying process, maximizing the values the patient treasured in life, and bringing comfort.

Guidelines 11 and 21 contain a wealth of material. Before discussing it, it would be useful to describe the experience of being desperately ill. For it is against such a background that Guideline 11 is relevant.

A common denominator amid the various effects of serious illness is the radical disruption of ordinary life. J. H. van den Berg notes: "The beginning of every serious illness is a halt. Normal life is at an end."[4] Renee C. Fox puts it this way:

> Illness is not just a biological "aspect". . . . Illness is also a disturbance in the psychological and social functioning of an individual. Particularly when his illness is a serious one, "being sick" greatly modifies the ordinary patterns of a man's existence. It removes him from the sphere of his normal social activities and sets him down in a "new world."[5]

This halt or removal from the sphere of one's normal activities can be accompanied by melancholy, confusion, anger, outrage, weakness, depression, or a host of other perplexing feelings. Alexander Solzhenitsyn notes:

> When melancholy sets in, a kind of invisible but thick and heavy fog invades the heart, envelops the body, constricting its very core. All we feel is this constriction, this haze around us. We don't even understand at first what it is that grips us.[6]

Disorientation is a common feature of many illnesses. Once again, Solzhenitsyn describes its basis very well:

> For thirty years she had been dealing with other people's illnesses. . . . During this time what she had worked out empirically for herself had become more and more indisputable, while in her mind medical theory grew increasingly coherent. . . .
> Then suddenly, within a few days, her own body had fallen out of this great, orderly system. It had struck the hard earth and was now like a helpless sack crammed with organs—organs which might at any moment be seized with pain and cry out. . . .

The course of her disease and her new place in the system of treatment had now become equally unrecognizable to her. As from today she ceased to be a rational guiding force in the treatment; she had become an unreasoning, resistent lump of matter.... Her world had capsized, the entire arrangement of her existence was disrupted.[7]

This collapse of one's ordinary world, when combined with physical weakness and a kaleidoscope of confusing and conflicting emotions most often leads to passivity and a sense of helplessness. Things are done to the patient. Drugs are prescribed for the patient. The patient eats when the system provides food. The patient often urinates and defecates in unaccustomed ways. This passivity is only deepened by the asymmetrical power relationship of physician and institution to patient. Renee Fox states it well:

Like all patients, the men of ward F–second were expected to entrust themselves to the physicians responsible for their care; to undergo the procedures that these physicians felt were necessary for the diagnosis and treatment of their conditions; to take the medications which had been prescribed for them; and, in general, to "follow the doctors' orders."

This patient passivity and helplessness is only deepened by the still-dominant Hippocratic principle: "I will [work] for the benefit of the sick according to my ability and judgment." An ethic built on this principle concentrates heavily on beneficence to the neglect of patient autonomy and creates very fertile soil for the practice of highly paternalistic medicine.

It is against this background that Guideline 11 insists that the patient is the primary decisionmaker and has the right to accept or reject medical treatment. This patient autonomy is rooted in the dignity of the person. Scrupulous respect for it is one key way of respecting the person.

By saying that the patient is the primary decisionmaker, Guideline 11 does not suggest that the physician and institution exist simply to respond to the patient's dictates or that the patient is the *only* decisionmaker; Guideline 11 does not support structural libertarianism. Many physicians believe they ought to be value-neutral. From a Catholic point of view this is simply false. (Indeed, it is increasingly admitted across a broad spectrum that value-free science is a myth.) It makes the physician a mere technologist. Physicians have consciences and institutions have chartered responsibilities that can at times clash with the values of the individual patient. In this sense, Guideline 11 immediately adds that "other secondary decisionmakers also have responsibilities."

Guideline 11 then makes explicit what is too often overlooked: health care decisions are not exclusively scientific judgments. They are choices based on one's beliefs and values. In other words, different people have different beliefs and values, and decisions about treatment must be in accord with these beliefs and values. Therefore, the treatment decision is a broadly human or moral judgment.

But what if the patient is incompetent? Guideline 11 underscores the responsibility of secondary decisionmakers. This is "normally" the next of kin (husband, wife, brother, sister, or children) because they are *presumed* to know the patient best and to be able to discuss his or her best interests. Where this is not the case a proxy (for example, a guardian *ad litem*) should be appointed by judicial intervention.

Guideline 11 deals clearly and concisely with one of the more confused areas of contemporary health care: decisions about the incompetent. Two questions arise in decisions about the incompetent: Who should make the decision? and On what basis should the decision be made? Answers to these questions were referred to as "confused areas." Two cases will make this clear.

The first instance is that of Joseph Saikewicz. In 1976 he was sixty-seven years old. He was mentally retarded, having the intelligence of a two-year-old (IQ of ten). Saikewicz communicated with grunts, groans, and gestures. He had been institutionalized since 1923 and in Belchertown State School since 1928.

On April 19, 1976, he was diagnosed as having acute myloblastic monocytic leukemia (excessive white blood cells). This involved enlargement of organs (spleen, lymph glands, bone marrow), internal bleeding, and eventually death. In 30 to 50 percent of such cases, chemotherapy produces a remission of from two to thirteen months, but the prognosis is poorer after age sixty. Without chemotherapy, the patient dies after several weeks or months.

Should Saikewicz receive such therapy? The Belchertown officials said yes. On April 26 they petitioned the probate court to appoint a guardian *ad litem* with authority for treatment decisions. On May 6 the guardian *ad litem* reported that "not treating is in his best interests." The probate court agreed on May 13. Saikewicz died on September 4 of bronchial pneumonia.

The probate court's decision was cautionarily appealed to the Massachusetts Supreme Court. Two questions were asked: Does the probate court have authority to order withholding of treatment in certain cases? and Was its judgment in the Saikewicz case correct?

On July 9, 1976 the Supreme Court answered in the affirmative to both questions and stated that its opinion would follow.

It did—on July 29, 1977. The court argued that there is a general right of self-determination based on human dignity. It is a general right only, since the state has interests that can prevail against it. Four were listed: the preservation of life, protection of the interests of innocent third parties (for example, children would suffer abandonment by a Jehovah's Witness refusing treatment), the prevention of suicide, the maintenance of the integrity of the medical profession.

The most important of these interests is clearly the preservation of life. But the Massachusetts Supreme Court noted: "The interest of the state in prolonging a life must be reconciled with the interest of the individual to reject the traumatic cost of that prolongation." Applied to Saikewicz, two interests were irrelevant (suicide and the protection of innocent third parties —for Saikewicz was himself abandoned). The other two did not override, for it is fully within accepted medical standards to withhold treatment at times. Moreover, in this case, life could have been only "briefly extended."

This analysis is based on the competent patient (self-determination). But what about the incompetent? Does a choice exist for them also? Must life-prolonging treatment *always* be ordered? The court asserted that a choice does exist: "To presume that the incompetent person must always be subjected to what rational and intelligent persons may decline is to downgrade the status of the incompetent person by placing a lower value on his intrinsic worth and vitality."[9]

How are the incompetent to exercise this right? The court replied: by a "substituted judgment," namely, what the incompetent would choose were he competent. Saikewicz would choose no treatment, for it is not in his best interest. Why? He had at best only a short time to live and the treatment would have inflicted painful and distressing side effects. These the competent can contextualize via their hope. Not so Saikewicz.

The court then turned to the procedure appropriate for withholding or withdrawing treatment from incompetents. In the case of Karen Quinlan, the New Jersey Supreme Court had entrusted the decision to Joseph Quinlan (Karen's father) in consultation with physicians and a badly so-called "ethics committee" (it was really a prognosis committee). The Massachusetts Supreme Court rejected this approach. It stated that questions of life and death require "a detached but passionate investigation and decision that forms the ideal on which the judicial branch of government was created." The decision is not to be entrusted to individuals or groups. Writing in *The Washington Post* Richard Knox noted:

> The new Massachusetts ruling essentially holds that issues of both with-
> holding and terminating critical care—for elderly stroke victims or cancer
> patients as well as for severely ill newborns—are matters for the probate
> courts to decide, not for the families, doctors, nurses, social workers,
> priests, committees, or anyone else.[10]

George Annas, assistant professor of law at Boston University School of
Medicine, agreed with the court. A correct resolution for incompetents, he
said,

> is more likely to come from a judicial decision after an adversary proceed-
> ing in which all interested parties have fully participated . . . than from
> individual decisions of the patient's family, the attending physician, an
> ethics committee, or all of these combined.[11]

For many reasons I disagree with that conclusion, as does Guideline 11,
if it is understood to apply to all incompetents. First of all, good consultation contains an adversary procedure. Caring nurses and physicians are
most often patient advocates. The Massachusetts decision attributes a prudence to probate judges that it denies to others. There is here an uninten-
tional but unmistakable judicial arrogance. These decisions are not exclusively medical or legal decisions; they are moral ones.

Second, by implication all incompetent patients must be kept on respirators until the probate judge says otherwise. Physicians are forced to start
treatment to find out whether they should. What happens to the patient in
the meantime? He or she could suffer as the legal machinery grinds into action. Those with clinical exposure know that conditions and prognoses
change. Must physicians return repeatedly to the probate court? If so, the
court becomes a cophysician.

Third, this ruling will simply intensify a new "vitalism"—a "never-say-
die" attitude and practice that is at odds with the cherished convictions of
many people about the meaning of life and death.

Finally, there is the sheer impracticality of the decision. There are hundreds of such cases daily. The courts, already overburdened, are incapable
of handling such cases promptly. Hospitals are likely to ignore the ruling,
thus undermining the integrity of the legal system and deepening the liability atmosphere of medical practice.

The second case is that of Brother Joseph Fox. Fox was an 83-year-old
member of the Society of Mary. On October 2, 1980 he underwent hernia
surgery. He experienced cardiorespiratory arrest and suffered diffuse cere-

bral and brain-stem anoxia. He was maintained on a respirator and the physician said he was in a "permanent vegetative state."

Reverend Philip K. Eichner, Fox's religious superior, after conferring with Fox's relatives, requested the removal of the respirator. Nassau Hospital refused. Eichner went to court. On December 6 Judge Robert Meade granted the relief.

Eichner argued that maintaining Fox on a respirator was an invasion of his constitutionally guaranteed right to privacy. He was relying on *Quinlan* and *Saikewicz*. Meade refused to pass on this. The right to privacy, he noted, is protected by the Fourteenth Amendment, which deals with restrictions on state actions. Some state action must occur before the constitutional right to privacy is invoked. Furthermore, the right to privacy is insufficiently defined and invites "unrestrained applications."

Meade appealed instead to the common-law notion of self-determination. There is such a right "which includes the right of a competent adult to refuse life-sustaining medical treatment." Fox, of course, could not exercise this right for himself. Eichner was seeking to do so for him, relying on the substituted-judgment doctrine in *Quinlan* and *Saikewicz*, but Meade rejected this. By its very nature the right to decline life-sustaining treatment can be exercised by the individual alone. Therefore, Meade rejected the substituted judgments in *Quinlan* and *Saikewicz* as involving a fiction: what they would have done had they been competent is not concludable in either case, in *Quinlan* for lack of evidence and in *Saikewicz* because he was never competent.

But Meade gave the relief because Fox had indicated his preference while he was still competent. Meade stated: "If Father Eichner, his committee, were to request the termination of the respirator, then that request would be the decision of Brother Fox which Father Eichner would merely pass on as a conduit. Unlike *Quinlan* and *Saikewicz*, no fiction is created nor is the judgment of Father Eichner substituted for that of Brother Fox."[12]

In other words, Meade granted relief only because the decision was that of Brother Fox. It was so only because Fox had seriously discussed the Karen Quinlan case and made his views clear ("none of that extraordinary stuff"). Any other analysis Meade sees as a substitued judgment which must be disallowed—at least as it is found in *Quinlan* and *Saikewicz*.

It is true that Meade was passing judgment only on the Fox case. But such decisions do get read by others. The implication is that the vast majority of incompetent patients will be unable to get off of respirators, either because they did not previously discuss the matter or there were no witnesses to the discussion.

Earlier, two questions were raised: Who makes the decision for incompetents and on what basis? The tendency of some courts is to answer that the basis is self-determination. If that is not possible, then the probate judge must make the decision.

In these decisions and others like them, there are two key notions that need clarification: substituted judgment and best interests.

Substituted Judgment

It should be clear that Joseph Saikewicz was never competent. Hence a substituted judgment (what he would do were he competent) is out of the question. Meade is correct in calling appeal to such a judgment a "fiction." But that suggests the wisdom of enlarging the notion of substituted judgment.

Edmund N. Santurri and William Werpehowski have suggested that we distinguish three different types of substituted judgment.[13]

First, there are "transmitted decisions." This refers to an explicitly articulated decision of the agent which is then conveyed by a medium external to the agent. This could be another person (proxy) or some other means (for example, the living will). Here there is no speculation about what the person would decide. The decision has been made but is conveyed by another. The Fox case is an example. Meade stated that there is no substituted judgment here. Strictly speaking, that is correct. But, as Santurri and Werpehowski note, there is a "substitutive function" and the notion of substituted judgment might be broadened to include it. In neither *Quinlan* nor *Saikewicz* can we speak of a transmitted decision. The concern to respect transmitted decisions involves respect for personal autonomy.

Second, there is the "hypothetical judgment"—what the person would do were that person competent. Basic to such a judgment is an assumption that the person had a least a rudimentary understanding of the alternatives. Without it, no preference can be determined. Thus, it is clear that there are insurmountable problems in using a hypothetical judgment in *Saikewicz*. Once again, hypothetical judgments respect the autonomy of incompetents because they recognize a prevailing value in self-chosen commitment.

Finally, there are "guardian judgments." These are objective assessments of what constitutes a person's best interests, all things considered. Such judgments bear no relation to respect for an incompetent's self-determination. They are in order precisely because self-determination is not possible.

A good example of a guardian judgment is the case of John Storar. Storar had a mental age of eighteen months. Since the age of five, he had lived in an institution for the mentally retarded. At 52 he was diagnosed as suffering from terminal cancer of the bladder. His seventy-seven-year-old mother, who was his guardian, initially approved of blood transfusions, but later asked that they be discontinued. Without them, Storar would die in two or three weeks. With them, he would die of cancer within six months.

Judge Wachtler rejected as "unrealistic" any attempt to determine what Storar "would want . . . were he competent." The court treated him as an infant and concluded that a guardian should not allow him to bleed to death. This is a guardian judgment with no appeal to autonomy. It was based simply in best interests.

Santurri and Werpehowski conclude that if respect for persons is to be interpreted exclusively in terms of respect for autonomy (as in *Saikewicz*), then guardian judgments violate respect for persons. It further means that incompetents like Storar and Saikewicz could not be treated as persons in medical judgments about them. That means that their best interests could not be served.

Best Interests

The concept of best interests is frequently used but rarely analyzed. In an excellent study, Edmund Pellegrino has noted that this concept has several components.[14] An ideal decision should attend to all of the components.

1. *Medical good.*   This refers to the effects of medical intervention on the natural history of the disease being treated, to what can be achieved by application of medical knowledge: cure, containment, prevention, amelioration, prolongation of life. This good can vary. For instance, the respirator could lead to complete recovery; or it could tide a patient over a crisis so that the underlying causes could be studied; or it can be used to discover whether the patient is terminal.

Pellegrino notes that there is a tendency for physicians to equate medical good with patient good. When that occurs, two fallacies may result. First, if any procedure *can* be done, it *ought* to be. All dimensions of patient good are conflated into medical good. Second, there is the expansion of medical good to include quality-of-life determinations. Then, if treatment of a defective newborn would result in a life "without meaningful relationships," it is not *medically* indicated. But, as Pellegrino correctly notes, this intermingling of goods exceeds medical competence. Whether a life is worth living is not a medical decision nor is it measurable by medical means.

2. *Patient preferences.*   The scientifically correct (medically good) decision must be placed within the context of the patient's life situation or value system. To be appropriate in this second sense, the choice must square with what the patient thinks worthwhile. Only the patient or his or her

proxy can determine whether ensuing life is worthwhile and whether one's belief system permits it or demands it.

3. *The good of the human as human.* This refers to the good proper to humans as humans. Pellegrino notes that this is philosophically debatable: among the various values associated with this good are freedom, rationality, consciousness, and the capacity for creativity. One thing is not debated: unique to humans is the very capacity to make choices, to set a life plan. This capacity is frustrated if choice is not free. To be treated as humans includes being accorded the dignity of choosing what we believe to be good. (I say "include" because self-determination does not exhaust the basis for respect for persons.) Therefore, all other things being equal, a treatment that preserves the capacity to choose is to be preferred to one that does not. In this sense it is in the patient's best interests.

4. *The good of last resort.*[15] This is the good that gathers all others, is their base and explanation. It gives life ultimate meaning. It will or should inform and explain patient preferences and life plans.

There are two noteworthy aspects of the good of last resort. First, it will differ among patients, depending on their belief systems. For example, the Orthodox Jew may regard every moment of life as precious, as absolute. For the Catholic, physical existence is relativized by the death-resurrection motif. The accumulation of minutes is not the Catholic criterion of dying well.

Second, with the always incompetent patient, it will be this good that will undergird the judgment of "best interests." Therefore judgments of best interests may differ. Reasonable persons may have differing theologies. For instance, with my beliefs, I could easily conclude that chemotherapy was not in Saikewicz's best interests. Someone else could disagree, and with plausibility, because of a different good of last resort.

Guideline 21 is an attempt to draw out concretely basic Catholic attitudes toward suffering and death. Guideline 20 had referred to suffering and dying as "a means of inner transformation to deeper life as well as a redemptive prayer for others." Pain and suffering will always remain a mystery; they will confuse, confound, and, at times, anger us. Why me? Why my mother? Why this useless tragedy? I remember standing at the bedside of Karen Quinlan, asking myself, in uncomprehending silence, similar questions.

Yet, without glorifying suffering, Catholic Christianity has always viewed it within a larger perspective—that of the redemptive process. Just as Christ suffered and died for us to enter his glory, so we who are "in the

Lord," who are inserted into the redemptive mystery, must expect that our growth "to deeper life" will share the characteristics of God's engendering deed in Christ. Catholic faith has, therefore, moved between trust and incomprehension. Michael Quoist has caught this beautifully:

> This afternoon I went to see a patient at the hospital.
> From pavilion to pavilion I walked, through that city of suffering,
>   sensing the tragedies hardly concealed by the brightly painted walls
>   and the flower-bordered lawns.
> I had to go through a ward; I walked on tiptoe, hunting for my patient.
>
> My eyes passed quickly and discreetly over the sick, as one touches a
>   wound delicately to avoid hurting.
> I felt uncomfortable,
> Like the noninitiated traveler lost in a mysterious temple,
> Like a pagan in the nave of a church.
> At the very end of the second ward I found my patient,
> And once there, I could only stammer. I had nothing to say.
>
> Lord, suffering disturbs me, oppresses me.
> I don't understand why you allow it.
> Why, Lord?
> Why this innocent child who has been moaning for a week, horribly
>   burned?
> This man who has been dying for three days and three nights, calling for
>   his mother?
> This woman with cancer who in one month seems ten years older?
> This workman fallen from his scaffolding, a broken puppet less than
>   twenty years old?
> This stranger, poor isolated wreck, who is one great open sore?
> This girl in a cast, lying on a board for more than thirty years?
> Why, Lord?
> I don't understand.
> Why this suffering in the world
>   that shocks,
>   isolates,
>   revolts,
>   shatters?
> Why this hideous suffering that strikes blindly, seemingly without cause,
> Falling unjustly on the good, and sparing the evil;
> Which seems to withdraw, conquered by science, but comes back in
>   another form, more powerful and more subtle?
> I don't understand.
> Suffering is odious and frightens me.
> Why thesè people, Lord, and not others?
> Why these, and not me?

Son, it is not I, your God, who have willed suffering; it is men.
They have brought it into the world in bringing sin,
Because sin is disorder, and disorder hurts.
There is for every sin, somewhere in the world and in time, a
    corresponding suffering.
And the more sins there are, the more suffering.

But I came, and I took all your sufferings upon me, as I took all your sins,
I took them and suffered them before you.
I transformed them, I made of them a treasure.
They are still an evil, but an evil with a purpose,
For through your sufferings, I accomplish Redemption.[16]

From the Christian point of view then, grave illness must be seen as an intensifying conformity to Christ. In this sense as the body weakens and is devastated, the strength of Christ is shared by those baptized into his death and resurrection. It is the Catholic conviction, therefore, that grave illness should be a time of grace, of the gradual shedding of the sinful self. This conviction takes concrete form in the sacrament of the anointing of the sick.

The understanding of the sacrament has had an interesting history. It is a matter of regrettable fact that all too often the administration of anointing of the sick is delayed until death is certain or, even worse, until it is instant (*articulum mortis*). Actually nothing of the sort is demanded by the provisions of canon law. Canon 1004 of the new code reads: "The anointing of the sick can be administered to any member of the faithful who, having reached the age of reason, begins to be in danger of death by reason of illness or old age." Misinterpretation of the meaning of danger plus a certain understandable reluctance to confront the patient with the gravity of his sickness has led to unfortunate delays in administering the anointing of the sick.

Revival of liturgical theology together with a laudable unrest in the face of improper delays has led increasingly to a modern emphasis away from *in extremis* administration of the anointing of the sick. This desirable shift in practical attitudes toward the sacrament has led many writers to refer to the anointing of the sick as the sacrament of the sick, not the sacrament of the dying. To others this opposition (sick versus dying) has appeared to represent an opposition of extremes. More accurately, they say, the anointing of the sick is the sacrament of the dangerously sick, of those whose sickness involves some danger. This is a middle course.

The "Constitution on the Liturgy" promulgated by Paul VI at the close of the second session of the Second Vatican Council has, it seems to me, adopted this middle course as a practical pastoral attitude. Paragraph 73 reads:

> "Extreme Unction" which may also and more fittingly be called "anointing of the sick" is not a sacrament for those only who are at the point of death. Hence, as soon as any one of the faithful begins to be in danger from sickness or old age, the fitting time for him to receive this sacrament has certainly arrived.[17]

This statement of the Constitution is a practical, pastoral statement. It represents the terminus of an historical process which witnessed different emphases in different eras. These emphases, of course, had a great effect on pastoral and homiletic attitudes. At those times when the sacrament was regarded as especially one for the sick, the theological and homiletic approach emphasized reinvigoration, restoration, and recovery. When it was viewed as especially a sacrament of the dying, the dominant theme was death, consecration of death, and anointing for glory.

The liturgical evidence up to the twelfth century presents the anointing of the sick as a sacrament of the sick. Then came the scholastic theologians and for them the sacrament meant anointing for glory, consecration of agony, and immediate preparation for entrance into glory. It was in the twelfth century that the name Extreme Unction originated. The scholastics drew the logical conclusion that the sacrament was to be received only when death was imminent. From Thomistic to pre-Tridentine times this emphasis was terribly exaggerated—to the point where the anointing of the sick was delayed until the recipient was all but clinically dead. Reformation and post-Reformation theologians felt pressured into the stoutest possible defense of purgatory and its pains, and so continued this emphasis.

Joseph Kern's classic *De Sacramento E. Unctionis* revived the anointing-for-glory emphasis and placed great stress on the remission of temporal punishment.[18] This sacrament-of-the-dying approach has found many modern followers. Yet there are those who reject Kern's thesis and its more current popularizations and wish to restore the anointing of the sick to what they call its proper place as the sacrament of the sick, with corresponding emphasis on the spiritually strengthening effects of the sacrament.

In summary, then, the early practice in the Church emphasized the healing powers of the sacrament, whereas systematic theology put the emphasis more on the sacrament as a final preparation for heaven. Both of these interpretations led to abuses, as P. Anciaux has shown.[19] During the earlier period anointing was too often reduced to a quasi-magical remedy to be administered for any ailment. Later the sacrament was delayed as long as possible and most Christians began to look upon it as a blessing for the dying or dead.[20] In modern times a proper balance has been found.

Just as suffering is viewed as transformative, so also is death. Guideline 21 reflects this very succinctly when it notes that the dying person "presents the health care team with one of its greatest challenges and opportunities. . . , to be with the dying and the family in a way which reproduces and mediates the fullest and final sense of Christ's healing love." This "being with" takes on meaning only when we attempt to understand death from a Christian perspective.

John Wright, S.J., describes the Christian perspective as follows:

> Sacred Scripture describes man's need of salvation in many ways. He is said to be in captivity or bondage, to be a slave, to be wandering astray, to be in debt, to be living according to the flesh (in the Pauline sense of creaturely weakness cut off from the divine strength), to be sick, to be in darkness, to be subject to futility. But all of these ways and many others are summed up in saying that sinful man is mortal, dwelling in the shadow of death, is, in fact, dead in sin. Death in these expressions does not mean exclusively either the material death of the body or the spiritual death of the soul but total death as it afflicts man's entire person. Salvation, then, must mean a transformation of man's mortal condition, a changing of death into life.
>
> God's determination to save man did not mean that He would erase death and pretend that man's sin had never happened. God's respect for created freedom and activity never allows Him to act as if some actual event had not occurred. The fact of man's sin remains and the consequences of that fact remain also. But God can change the internal meaning of those consequences, and provided only man is willing, thereby make those consequences work for man's ultimate well-being, instead of for his ultimate destruction. This change cannot be simply a different way of looking at death from the outside, nor an arbitrary connection of death with certain beneficent effects to which it bears in itself no inner relationship. Rather, the very nature of death must be changed so that it leads to God and life, rather than away from Him to everlasting ruin.[21]

This inner transformation of death was achieved by Jesus Christ. As Wright words it:

> The gift of Himself in death was accepted by the Father, who raised Him from the dead and filled Him with the undying life of the Holy Spirit. Death is swallowed up in victory. In Christ its meaning has been totally transformed. It no longer means simply man's rebellion against God; it is also now a sign of the presence of God's saving love in the world.[22]

Thus the death of the Christian is viewed as the fulfillment of the life of grace, the completion of the sacraments, as a step toward the coming of God's kingdom, as a sharing of one side of Christ's paschal mystery. As such, it is clearly the decisive moment in each person's life. For it is viewed as fixing for all eternity a person's intention. As this moment the soul ceases to act in a fundamentally changeable way. The "period of probation" is over.

How is that to be understood? There is no unanimous agreement among Catholic theologians. Some propose a theory of "final option," a perfectly free act wherein at death one definitively and irrevocably chooses either to ratify the life one has led or to reject it.

There are real problems with such a theological understanding of death. Perhaps first and foremost is the lack of evidence in Scripture for such a decision on which everything depends. Quite the contrary. "We must all appear before the tribunal of Christ in order to receive good and evil, according to what each has done in the body."[23]

More concretely, one can argue that a "final option" theory denies the grace of forgiveness.[24] Where traditional teaching says that every mortal sin is *of itself* definitive and that it is provisional only by virtue of the free grace of divine forgiveness, the final-option theory says that every sin before death is *of itself* only provisional because it arises out of lesser insight and freedom than is required for definitive decision. Therefore the possibility of conversion remaining to the mortal sinner is not seen in this theory as grounded in the forgiving grace of God, but in the imperfection of every free self-disposition of earthly man. This means that the final-option theory must render the grace of forgiveness superfluous. Why? Because looking at himself and his acts, the "mortal sinner" is certain in advance that he will have the opportunity to convert to God. He is certain of this because he knows that he was able to dissociate himself only provisionally from God and therefore did so only provisionally. God, therefore, could dissociate himself only provisionally from the sinner. Because the sinner's decision was not definitive, God simply must offer himself again as salvation, not from grace but from justice. In summary, the sin-unto-death as absolutely irrevocable is unforgivable; mortal sin prior to this, as not definitive, needs no forgiveness purely from grace.

Bruno Schüller advances this argument from a slightly different perspective. In the New Testament the grace of forgiveness is seen as that given against one's deserts. Forgiveness by grace means that a man has brought his salvation history to an end. He is a definitively damned person, but God makes a radically new start. Forgiveness by grace is the conversion of the end into a radically new start. Therefore it can only become a reality after a genuine end has occurred. Since, therefore, the final-option theory denies to man the possibility of putting a real end to his history with God during earthly life, it implicitly denies that God needs to place any new beginning in his history with man. And this is to render forgiveness as we know it in the New Testament superfluous.

According to Schüller, then, mortal sin and sin-unto-death are, insofar as they depend on the sinner alone, irreparable and decisive. The qualitative difference between the two depends not on the sinner's self-disposition, but on a radically gratuitous act of God. To say otherwise, as the final-option theory must, is to attack this forgiveness.

Schüller's second argument is that the only-provisional-mortal-sin is really slight sin. The defenders of the final-option theory believe that mortal sins remain mortal sins even when man turns only "provisionally" from God in this life. Schüller denies this. Each act, he argues, receives its special character from that to which it turns (*actus specificatur ab objecto*). From the fact that in mortal sin man turns from God his last end we can conclude what kind of freedom must be present in mortal sin. Precisely because the last end is that which is sought before and in all, mortal sin can only be a turning from God as last end if man, insofar as it depends on him, totally and definitively engages himself in a free decision. But totality and definitiveness are precisely the qualities absent in any sin but the sin-unto-death in the final-option theory. Therefore these sins simply cannot be mortal.

In spite of these disagreements about the *theological* understanding of death among contemporary Catholics, the areas of agreement should not be overlooked. Wright summarizes them as follows:

> Although there is a real difference of opinion between these groups of theologians on the nature of the act of the soul in the moment of death, it would be a mistake to exaggerate this difference. Both agree that this act depends profoundly and inescapably upon the prior choices made while the soul is in the state of union with the body. If one position says that these prior choices do not wholly necessarily determine this act from within, this is not said to encourage sinners to put off their repentance and plan to fix things up at that last instant of freedom, but to make a man unequivocally assume full responsibility for the answer he makes to God's grace. Both agree, too, that in this act man becomes definitively himself, and that in the moment his preparation is joined intrinsically to divine fulfillment or to the awful emptiness of sin that remains forever. Both agree, finally, that the state that follows death does not derive its essential immutability from an extrinsic, free decree of God, but from the very nature of death and the activity elicited by the soul in this moment. Death and eternity hang upon mortal life and time.[25]

It is against the background of this discussion that Guideline 21 draws its more concrete ethical conclusions. The burden-benefit criterion for the acceptance or rejection of medical treatment is that proposed by the Sacred Congregation for the Doctrine of the Faith. Indeed, the very language ("secure a precarious and burdensome prolongation of life") is its language.

The directive about pain relievers ("even if a side effect is the shortening of life") is drawn from Pius XII. It should provide support and security to those practitioners—and they are too many—who are reluctant for moral and possibly legal reasons to provide adequate pain relief.

PRENATAL LIFE

15. *Since all individual human life deserves respect and protection, every reasonable effort must be made to nourish, support, and protect life in the womb. Thus, abortion has been rejected by the Church in the vast majority of instances as a violation of the respect due to nascent life.*

Guideline 15 proposes an attitude (respect) and a general practice (protection). This general practice is then further defined as an effort to "nourish, support, and protect." These notions are close but not necessarily identical. *Nourish* suggests a healthy nutritional regime and supposes the absence of substances likely to be harmful to the fetus (cigarettes, alcohol, harmful drugs). *Support* may be read to mean any kind of intervention (for example, in utero surgery, special nutrition) aimed at alleviating fetal distress or correcting fetal pathology. *Protect* in this context refers to the claim of nascent life not to be made the subject of distressing or dangerous nontherapeutic experimentation, and, above all, not to be aborted. Guideline 15 summarizes the Catholic attitude toward abortion as morally wrong "in the vast majority of instances."

Catholic convictions on abortion developed over the centuries. The debates and struggles that were part of this process are splendidly detailed by John R. Connery, S.J., in his historical study *Abortion: The Development of the Roman Catholic Perspective*.[26] What emerges from Connery's study is the fact that the ethical history of abortion is the history of an evaluation. What has that evaluation been? Over the centuries, some theologians, because of the biological knowledge available to them, spoke of three types of abortion: prevention of conception, abortion of an inanimate fetus, abortion of an animated fetus. Still others felt that all interventions into the life-giving process were homicides. Others argued that the evacuation of a non-animated fetus was permissible to save the mother's life, for the inanimate fetus was not yet a human being. Some contended that abortion even of an inanimate fetus was immoral, either as imperfect homicide or as misuse of *semen conceptum*.

As time went on, many of these qualifications vanished and obscurities diminished. Beneath these debates and developments, one finds an evaluation of prenatal life that yielded it to very few competing interests—what John Noonan calls "an almost absolute value."[27]

The late André Hellegers, M.D., is surely correct, then, when he insists that the fundamental question (not the only question, nor necessarily the most sensitive) in contemporary debates on abortion is: "When shall we attach value to human life?"[28] The basic question is not "When does life begin?" It is: "When does dignity begin?" Of the Supreme Court's 1973 ruling (*Roe v. Wade*) Hellegers notes:

> They have used terms like "potential life" trying to say that life wasn't there, when the reason for saying that life wasn't there was because they didn't attach any value to it. The abortion issue is fundamentally a value issue, not a biological one.

Has this evaluation changed in recent years? Not if papal and hierarchical statements are any indication. The Second Vatican Council noted that "from the moment of conception life must be guarded with the greatest care, while abortion and infanticide are unspeakable crimes."[29]

In the wake of the 1973 Supreme Court decision on abortion, many other countries began considering liberalization of their laws. This provided the occasion for a stream of papal and episcopal pronouncements. Since their context was that of threatened or actual liberalization of abortion law, there is a decided though far from exclusive emphasis on the relation of morality and law. Just a few statements will serve our purposes here.

Pope Paul VI, in an allocution to Italian jurists, noted that the state's protection of human life should begin at conception, "this being the beginning of a new human being."[30] This is an emphasis that appears in nearly all the national episcopal statements.

When relating abortion to women's liberation, Pope Paul insisted that true liberation is found in the vocational fulfillment of motherhood. There follows an extremely interesting analysis of the pertinence of relationships to human dignity and rights:

> In such a vocation there is implicit and called to concretization the first and most fundamental of the relations constitutive of the personality—the relation between this determined new human being and this determined woman, as its mother. But he who says *relation* says *right*; he who

says fundamental relation says *correlation between a right and an equally fundamental duty*; he who says fundamental human relationship says a universal human value, worthy of protection as pertaining to the universal common good, since every individual is before all else and constitutively *born of a woman.*[31]

If I read him correctly, Paul VI was insisting that the relationship constitutive of the personality and generative of rights and duties is not basically and primarily at the psychological or experienced level—a point I shall touch on later.

The Belgian bishops make this very same point.[32] Relationships—and by this they obviously mean experienced relationships—important as they are, are not the sources of the dignity and rights of the nascent child. Rather, the source is the personality in the process of becoming. They cite *Abortus Provocatus*, a study issued by the Center of Demographic and Family Studies of the Belgian Ministry of Health:

> There is no objective criterion for establishing, in the gradual process of development, a limit between "nonhuman" life and "human" life. In this process each stage is the necessary condition for the following and no moment is "more important," "more decisive," or "more essential" than another.[33]

Therefore they are puzzled at the fact that at the very time we are eliminating discrimination between sexes and among races and social classes, we are admitting at the legal level another form of discrimination based on the moment, more or less advanced, of life.

As for the law itself, the Belgian hierarchy is convinced that liberalized abortion law does not solve the real problems. Indeed, by seeming to, it leads society to neglect efforts on other fronts to get at the causes of abortion. Therefore they are opposed to removal of abortion from the penal code, because such removal would, among other things, imply the right to practice abortion and would put in question one of the essential foundations of our civilization: respect for human life in all forms.

The Swiss bishops, after noting with other national hierarchies that God alone is the judge of conscience and that no one has the right to judge other persons, put great emphasis on corporate responsibility for the abortion situation.[34] Those who neglect the social measures for family protection, for aid to single women, etc., are more culpable than those who have abortions.

The bishops of Quebec echoed many of these same points and made it clear that what is at stake is the very idea on which our civilization is built: the conviction that all persons are equal, whether young or old, rich or poor, sick or well, etc.[35] They associated themselves with all people who seek truly human solutions through establishment of a more just and humane society.

The German episcopate, after noting that protection of human life is an "absolutely fundamental principle," registered its opposition to the liberalization before the Bundestag.[36] Not only is the legislation morally unacceptable, but it will not solve the alleged difficulties it is supposed to solve. In the course of this interesting statement, the bishops turn to the relation of morality and law. Clearly, not every moral imperative should be in the penal code (for example, prohibitions of envy, ingratitude, or egoism). But where the rights of others are at stake, the state cannot remain indifferent:

> Its primordial duty is to protect the right of the individual, to assure the common good, to take measures against the transgressions of right and violations of the common good, if necessary by means of penal law.

In doing this, the state becomes a *constitutional* state.

But legislation is not enough. The difficulties leading to abortion must be overcome by other measures. It is here that genuine reform ought to occur. And in undertaking these reforms, the federal republic becomes a *social* state:

> It is only when the state is disposed to recognize the principle according to which no social need, whatever it be, can justify the killing of a human being before birth, that is merits the name of social state. It is only when the state is disposed to protect the right to life of a human being before birth and to punish violations of this right, that it merits the name of constitutional state.[37]

Only within these parameters and on these conditions should legislators withhold penal sanctions for conflict cases—cases that ought to be precisely determined in law.

Some years ago the Catholic Conference of German Bishops and the Protestant Council of the Evangelical Church produced a joint statement on abortion.[38] The most remarkable thing about the document is its common endorsement by the leadership of the vast majority of Christians, Catholic and non-Catholic, in Germany. Once again there is insistence on the fact that a social state will approach abortion reform positively, that is, in terms that attempt to reorder social relationships in such a way that pregnant women receive the type of support that will prevent their seeking abortion as the only way out of difficult circumstances. The bishops stress the fact that no society can long exist when the right to life is not acknowledged and protected:

> The right to life must not be diminished, neither by a judgment on the value or lack thereof of an individual life, nor by a decision on when life begins or ends. All decisions that touch human life can only be oriented to the service of life.

The document resolutely rejects the legalization of abortion in the first three months (*Fristenregelung*) as a form of abortion reform. Rather, the task of the lawmaker is to identify those conflict situations in which interruption of pregnancy will not be punished (*straflos lassen*). By this wording the document insists that the moral law is not abrogated by legal tolerance but it remains to guide individual decisions in exceptional situations where the state decides not to punish abortion. Throughout, the document puts emphasis on the fact that positive law regulating abortion is rooted not merely in considerations of utility and party politics, but also in basic human values (*Grundwerte menschlichen Zusammenlebens*). This is an excellent pastoral statement on all counts.

The Permanent Council of the French Episcopate calls attention to the difference between legislation and morality.[39] The task of the legislator is to see how the common good is best preserved in the circumstances. But in drawing up legislation, the government will necessarily express a certain concept of the person; for this reason the bishops feel impelled to speak up. Recalling that abortion, no matter how safe and clean it is, always represents a personal and collective human defeat, the bishops remind the legislators that in widening the possibilities for abortion they risk respect for human life, open the door for further extensions, and consecrate radical ruptures among sexuality, love, and fecundity. Ultimately, the remedy for the problem of widespread clandestine abortion in France is neither legal constraints nor liberalization. Women tempted to abort must experience, really and personally, the fact that they are not alone in their distress. Any reform of abortion law must provide for this.

The statement of the Administrative Committee of the National Conference of Catholic Bishops of the United States in response to the Supreme Court's *Wade* and *Bolton* decisions is the strongest, and in this sense the most radical, episcopal statement I have ever encountered.[40] After detailing the Court's assignation of prenatal life to nonpersonhood, the pastoral states: "We find that this majority opinion of the Court is wrong and is entirely contrary to the fundamental principles of morality." The document continues: "Laws that conform to the opinion of the Court are immoral laws, in opposition to God's plan of creation. . . ." After citing the fundamental character of the right to life as guaranteed in the Declaration of Independence and buttressed in the Preamble to the Constitution, the bishops conclude that "in light of these reasons, we reject the opinion of the United States Supreme Court as erroneous, unjust, and immoral." While the statement contains no protracted discussion on the relation of law and morality, it is clear that the American bishops utterly reject the implied doctrine of the Court on the question.

Even this brief survey probably justifies the conclusion of Michael J. Walsh, S.J., that we have an "impressive example of the magisterium in action."[41] It would be useful to list the major themes of this sprawling papal and episcopal literature. I see them as follows:

1.   There is total unanimity in the recent teaching of the Pope and bishops on the right to life from conception. Furthermore, as Philippe Delhaye points out,[42] there is the pronounced consciousness that this teaching is the fulfillment of the commission received by Christ to teach and witness to the constant teaching of the Church.

2.   There is repeated emphasis on the fact that we are dealing with a fundamental value, one at the very heart of civilization. The documents generally place the fight against abortion in the larger context of respect for life at all stages and in all areas.

3.   It is the task of civil society to protect human life from the very beginning.

4.   Human life is a continuum from the beginning. As Walsh puts it, "Essential continuity of a human being from conception to death is the presupposition of every episcopal argument."[43] In light of this we encounter terms such as "person in the process of becoming." And to this individual there is repeatedly ascribed the *droit de naître*, as Pope Paul put it, a relatively recent rendering of the more classical right to life.

5.   The protection provided for this *personne en devenir* must be both legal and social. With regard to the law, there is the practically unanimous conviction that legalization of abortion on a broad scale will not solve the many problems associated with abortion, but will rather bring further devastating personal and social evils, particularly through miseducation of consciences. Beyond that, the pastorals are rather reserved in their demands about legislation, except for the American statement, which Delhaye regards as *assez dur*. By *social protection* I refer to the unanimous and strongly stated conviction of the episcopates that we do

much more, personally and societally, to get at the causes of abortion. If there is a single major emphasis in all of the documents, it is this.

6. In arguing their case for respect for nascent life and for its protection through public policy, the hierarchies suit the argument to the local situation, as Walsh notes.[44] For instance, the Americans appeal to American legal traditions and the declaration of the United Nations. The Scandinavians, in opposing further liberalization, are deeply concerned to protect individuals against coercion.

7. The statements generally note that their teaching is not specifically Catholic, though the Church has always upheld it and though it can be illumined, enriched, and strengthened by theological sources.

8. While urging the teaching clearly and unflinchingly, the bishops manifest a great compassion for individuals in tragic circumstances and a refusal to judge these individuals. On the other hand, there is a rather persistent severity toward society in general, whose conditions so often render new births difficult or psychologically insupportable.

As a conclusion to this survey of contemporary thinking it would be useful to cite the remarkable pastoral letter of Bishops Eric Grasar and John Brewer, of the Diocese of Shrewsbury, England:

> We recognize that, for one reason or another, a pregnancy can cause a problem, distress, shame, despair to some mothers. Perhaps in our concern to uphold the sanctity of life, we have failed to show sufficient practical concern for the mother-to-be who feels herself in an intolerable situation. That is all over. The Diocese of Shrewsbury publicly declares its solemn guarantee. It is this: Any mother-to-be, Catholic or non-Catholic, is guaranteed immediate and practical help, if, faced with the dilemma of an unwanted pregnancy, she is prepared to allow the baby to be born and not aborted. This help includes, if she wishes, the care for her baby after birth. All the resources of the diocese are placed behind this pledge.[45]

At this point, several notes should be added to this chronicle. First, there is the distinction made by John XXIII and repeated by Vatican II between the substance of a teaching and its formulation at a given time in history. Karl Rahner says the same thing when he distinguishes between "a truth in itself and in its abiding validity" and its "particular historical formulation."[46] We know that at any given time our formulations—being the product of limited persons, with limited insight, and with imperfect philosophical and linguistic tools—are only more or less adequate to the substance of our convictions. It is the task of theology constantly to question and challenge these formulations in an effort to reduce their inadequacy.

How does this work out when applied to abortion? As human beings we know deep down (and with powerful supportive warrants from our belief that all persons are unique and equal before our heavenly Father) that human life is sacred, that no person may play God with regard to another. Yet we also know from experience that there are tragic instances of conflict, instances where we must sacrifice life to maintain our grasp on the very values we adhere to and treasure. Throughout our history we have attempted to provide for these instances as well as to contain them by correcting the conditions that lead to them. "No *direct* killing of an *innocent* person" is the rule we have developed to state the exceptions and to contain them.

Applying this to the abortion situation, several popes have stated that direct abortion is never permissible, even to save the life of the mother. Thus in the classic if rare case where the options are two (do nothing and both mother and nonviable child die; abort and save the only life that can be salvaged) it was concluded: "better two deaths than one murder." Almost no one would support that conclusion today. Some would argue that in such a case the abortion is indirect. Others would say that it is direct but morally permissible as the only life-saving, life-serving alternative available. The Belgian hierarchy, in its pastoral on abortion, summarized the matter as follows:

> The moral principle which ought to govern the intervention can be formulated as follows: Since two lives are at stake, one will, while doing everything possible to save both, attempt to save one rather than to allow two to perish.[47]

The only point I am making here is that our formulations of behavioral norms are only more or less adequate, and for this reason are inherently revisable. The fact that some theological formulations have been thought useful by the magisterium of the Church does not change this state of affairs. Historical consciousness has made us freshly aware of the fact that it is our onerous theological task to continue to test the validity of theological formulations, even some very hallowed ones. If we do not, we become imprisoned by words and commit the ever fresh *magnalia Dei* to unwarranted risks.

It is clear that the basic evaluation of prenatal life has come to us wrapped in a variety of formulations: direct and indirect abortion, immediate ensoulment and delayed ensoulment, fetus as aggressor, the prevalence of certain rights over doubtful rights, etc.

What is the substance of the classical moral position? Distinguishing the abiding substance from its changeable formulation is a tricky and difficult business—even, it would seem, an arrogant one. At a certain point one has to assume the posture of a person standing over history and filtering out the limitations of others when one is at least knee-deep in historical limitations oneself.

With that caution, I would like to repeat and expand in three statements the substance of the classical Christian moral position in our time.

1. Human life as a basic gift and good, the foundation for the enjoyment of all other goods, may be taken only when doing so is the only life-saving and life-serving alternative, or only when doing so is, all things considered (not just numbers), the lesser evil. I have said here "human life," not the "human person," for the word *person* only muddies the moral discussion. *Person*, as Albert Outler notes, is a code word for a self-transcending, transempirical reality.[48] Self-transcendence is not, contrary to the notions or wishes of so many, a part of the organism. It is the organism as oriented to its self-transcending matrix. I have said "life-saving and life-serving" for two reasons. First, not every life-saving action is life-serving. For example, some actions could, while saving lives, actually and simultaneously undermine other basic goods in a way that would be a disservice to life itself by attacking an associated value. Second, it seems to me that the exceptions historically tolerated (for example, ectopic pregnancies) fit this general category.

2. By "human life" is meant human life from fertilization or at least from the time at or after which it is settled whether there will be one or two distinct human beings (this phrase is Ramsey's). There are phenomena in the preimplantation period that generate evaluative doubts about the claims the fetus at this stage makes, at least in some cases. I refer to twinning, the number of spontaneous abortions, the possibility of recombination of two fertilized ova into one (chimeras), the time of the appearance of the primary organizer. These phenomena may create some problems. But we must remember that the only thing that stands between an eight-cell embryo in a petri dish and Louise Brown is a uterine home for two-hundred sixty-six days. I find it revealing that Louise Brown is referred to as the "test-tube *baby*." The answer to the question, "Where did Louise Brown begin?" is clearly "In the petri dish, if *baby* means anything." We did not say "test-tube tissue." When in doubt one ought to favor life—but I think not always. But more of this shortly.

3. For an act to be life-saving and life-serving, to be the lesser evil (all things considered), there must be at stake human life or its moral equivalent, a good or a value comparable to life itself. This is not what the traditional formulations say, but it is where the corpus of teachings on life-taking lead (for example, the issues of a just war and of capital punishment). For instance, if human beings may go to war and take human life to defend their freedom against an enemy, something is being said about human freedom compared with life. I realize that at a certain level—the theoretical and philosophical—life and liberty cannot be compared, as apples and oranges cannot. But in daily life we somehow manage to resolve this incommensurability in many areas. We choose to smoke or to drink or to eat creamy butter for enjoyment's sake at the risk of a shortened life. We elect a heart bypass operation to relieve oppressive and continuous chest pains, although we know the operation is still being investigated and may itself kill us. We choose a contemplative or a more active career for ourselves.

In each of these instances it is not inaccurate to say that we somehow manage to weigh incommensurables, to overcome indeterminacy. As philosopher Donald Evans has been known to say: Such compromises are a part of everyday morality, but they raise serious problems for ethical theory, for their logic and rationale are obscure. So we may grant with philosopher W. D. Ross that we are faced with great difficulties when we try to compare good things of very different types. But I would suggest that the difficulties are not insuperable. I make this very slight opening in fear and trembling because it is made in a world and at a time where it can be terribly misused and misunderstood. If that is a serious danger in our time, then our task is to develop controls and exception-stoppers. But I have known cases where failure to terminate a pregnancy has resulted in complete and permanent loss of freedom for the mother (who goes insane). We take life to preserve our freedom, do we not? "Give me liberty or give me death" resonates with all of us, though there are still some who would rather be "red than dead"— because, I suspect, they think they will really have their liberty after all.

I have presented at least, and perhaps at best, a defensible account of the substance of the Catholic community's evaluation of nascent life over the centuries. It is an evaluation I share. I want to make three points about the notion of evaluation. First, evaluation is a complex concept, involving many dimensions of human insight and judgment. It cannot be reduced simply to rational arguments or religious dogma. Persons with profound religious faith often make judgments that coincide with those of a genuine humanism. Having said that, I would add, however, that the best way to state why I share the traditional evaluation is that I can think of no persuasive arguments that limit the sanctity of human life to extrauterine life. In other words, arguments that justify abortion seem to me equally to justify infanticide—and more.

Second, by saying I share the evaluation, I do not mean to suggest that all problems are solved. They are not. For instance, the moral relevance of the distinction between direct and indirect abortion remains a theoretical problem of the first magnitude. I am inclined to agree with John Noonan, Bruno Schüller, Denis O'Callaghan, and, most recently, Susan Teft Nicholson that the distinction is not of crucial moral significance. For instance, O'Callaghan wrote:

> If it was honest with itself, it [the scholastic tradition] would have admitted that it made exceptions where these depended on chance occurrence of circumstances rather than on free human choice. In other words, an exception was admitted when it would not open the door to more and more exceptions, precisely because the occurrence of the exception was determined by factors of chance outside of human control.[49]

He gives intervention into ectopic pregnancy as an example. The casuistic tradition, he believes, accepted what is in principle an abortion because it posed no threat to the general position, though this tradition felt obliged to rationalize this by use of the double effect. Ectopic pregnancy, as a relatively rare occurrence and one independent of human choice, does not lay the way open to abuse.

In her recent study *Abortion and the Roman Catholic Church*, Susan Teft Nicholson has suggested that abortion might be reconceptualized. If it is viewed mainly as a killing intervention, certain conclusions will be drawn. If it is conceptualized above all as a withdrawal of maternal assistance, different questions arise—and possibly different answers. Thus this question comes up: Is a woman bound (heroically) to provide assistance (nourishment, etc.) when a pregnancy is the result of rape?[50] I shall not discuss this issue here except to say that Nicholson raises legitimate questions.

The third point to be made about this evaluation is its historical and theological basis. I have already cited Albert Outler on this matter, but his words deserve repetition here:

> One of Christianity's oldest traditions is the sacredness of human life as an implication of the Christian convictions about God and the good life. If all persons are equally the creatures of the one God, then none of these creatures is authorized to play God toward any other. And if all persons are cherished by God, regardless of merit, we ought also to cherish each

other in the same spirit. This was the ground on which the early Christians rejected the prevalent Greco-Roman codes of sexuality in which abortion and infanticide were commonplace. Christian moralists found them profoundly irreligious and proposed instead an ethic of compassion (adopted from their Jewish matrix) that proscribed abortion and encouraged "adoption."[51]

Thus the tradition has based the value of human life in God's special and costly love for each individual—for fetal life, infant life, senescent life, disabled life, captive life, enslaved life, and, most of all, unwanted life. These evaluations can be and have been shared by people outside the Christian tradition, of course. But Christians have particular warrants for resisting any cultural callousing of them.

Contemporary problems will always provoke doubts and questions and give rise to ambiguity. The Catholic tradition may well have some unfinished agenda and it would be counterproductive to the overall health of the position to leave this agenda unfinished or to sweep it under the carpet. I see three problem areas.

The first is, as was noted above, the status of the preimplanted embryo. There are phenomena in this period that raise evaluative doubts (twinning, possible recombination of fertilized ova, spontaneous wastage, hydatidiform moles, etc.). For instance, Karl Rahner has written that the traditional presupposition that an individual person comes into existence at fertilization is now "exposed to positive doubts." He continues:

> Will today's moral theologians still have the courage to maintain this presupposition as the basis of many of his moral theological statements, when faced with the knowledge that 50 percent of all fertilized female cells never succeed in becoming attached to the womb? Will he be able to accept that 50 percent of all "human beings"—real human beings with "immortal" souls and an eternal destiny—will never get beyond this first stage of human existence?[52]

Such considerations lead to the question: Are there not phenomena here that cast doubt on the validity of the term "termination of *pregnancy*" when applied to the preimplantation period? It is for this reason that Guideline 16 notes that

> treatment options . . . have important moral dimensions, some of which (prevention of implantation) are the subject of controversy in the Church. Health care institutions should be aware of these discussions and devise their policies in the light of them.

Practically speaking this suggests that prevention of implantation is not clearly wrong in such emergency situations.

Second, there is anencephaly. Does the anencephalic fetus possess a sufficient biological substratum to justify its inclusion among those morally protected against abortion? Bernard Häring originally raised this question in a different context. He proposed it in conjunction with the opinion that hominization of nascent life should be related to the development of the cerebral cortex; for it is the cerebral cortex that constitutes the biological substratum for personal life.[53] One need not hold *that* theory to propose that anencephalic beings are not fully protectable (against termination) individuals.

Finally, there is the instance of rupture of the membranes. If nature has started a process (with extremely low fetal survival expectation and rather high incidence of serious maternal infection in attempting to bring the fetus to term), does human completion of this process deserve the rejection implied in the term "abortion"? I raise these as questions for those concerned to protect fetal life but not to expand that protection deductively in a way harmful to the overall health of the position.

Marginal questions such as these, as well as two extreme emergency cases (ectopic pregnancy and cancerous uterus), are envisaged in Guideline 15 when it words its summary of Catholic tradition with "in the vast majority of instances."

One of the most interesting and divisive problems for the Catholic community is relating its convictions about fetal life to public policy. When the Supreme Court in 1973 handed down its historic decisions on abortion (*Roe v. Wade, Doe v. Bolton*), the administrative committee of the National Conference of Catholic Bishops rejected these decisions as "erroneous, unjust, and immoral."[54] Ever since that time there has been a vigorous effort to overturn the decisions, and Catholics have played a major role in this effort. But the relationship of moral conviction to public policy has not been a matter of unanimity. (The names of Robert Drinan, S.J., and Agnes Mary Mansour are the symbols of this problem. Drinan is now out of public life; Mansour is still in—but out of religious life.)

The abortion debate has raised the more general problem for the Catholic community of moral pluralism and public policy. Specifically, what is to be done at the policy level when people disagree on the moral level that is the basis of the policy? The very statement of the question rightly supposes that there is *some* relationship between morality and public policy. The statement that "you cannot and should not legislate morality" is a very dangerous half-truth. We do it all the time. Every civilized society has rules about homicide. The basic question is, *What* morality ought we legislate?

American opinion is divided on this matter. Indeed, the division is so heated that there now prevails a dialogue of the deaf on the matter. In the process, the very relationship of morality and law has been obscured.

I noted that there is *some* relationship between morality and legality. That is, what is good law or good public policy depends to some extent on morality. Concretely, if fetal life is regarded as disposable tissue, clearly abortion ought not be on the penal code at all, except to protect against irresponsible and dangerous tissue-scrapers. If, however, fetal life is to be regarded as human life, then there is the possibility that taking such life should be on the penal code.

Morality and public policy are related but distinct. They are related because morality is concerned with the rightness and wrongness of human conduct. Public policy has an inherently moral character due to its roots in existential human ends or goals. The welfare of the community (the proper concern of law) cannot be unrelated to what is judged promotive or destructive to individual human beings, to what is morally right or wrong.

Morality and public policy are distinct because an individual's actions are the proper concern of society only when they have ascertainable consequences for the maintenance and stability of society. Americans often forget this as they conflate public policy into their own moral convictions. The conclusion to many moral arguments is: "There 'oughta' be a law."

A key question, then, is this: What morally wrong actions affect the welfare of the community in a way that demands legislation? The famous Wolfenden Report distinguishes between crime and sin, between the private act and its public manifestation. But that is inadequate. What is done in private (outside of public scrutiny) is not necessarily a private act. Rather, the proper criterion is what we may call feasibility. All actions that have ascertainable public consequences for the maintenance and stability of society are legitimate matters of concern to society. They *can* be on the penal code.

But it is feasibility that tells us whether they *should be* on the penal code. Let me call to witness three authors in an attempt to illustrate this concept. Feasibility is:

> . . . that quality whereby a proposed course of action is not merely possible but practicable, adoptable, depending on the circumstances, cultural ways, attitudes, traditions of a people, etc. . . . any proposal of social legislation which is not feasible in terms of the people who are to adopt it is simply not a plan that fits man's nature as concretely experienced.[55]

> . . . a moral condemnation regards only the evil itself, in itself. A legal ban on an evil must consider what Saint Thomas calls its "own possibility."

That is, will the ban be obeyed, at least by the generality? Is it enforceable against the disobedient? Is it prudent to undertake the enforcement of this or that ban, in view of the possibility of harmful effects in other areas of social life? Is the instrumentality of coercive law a good means for the eradication of this or that social vice? And, since a means is not a good means if it fails to work in most cases, what are the lessons of experience in the matter?[56]

One cannot conclude . . . that because the state does not penalize some action it is not morally wrong. All one can infer is that it was not judged to be harmful to the community, *or if it was judged harmful, the harm was less than that which would result from prohibitive legislation.*[57]

The heart of the policy question is the moral evaluation of the fetus. The very rightness or wrongness whose legal possibility is under discussion is the object of doubt and controversy. We can identify at least three general moral positions. First, fetal life is living but disposable tissue. Second, fetal life is human life making claims on us, but claims that are overridden by a rather broad class of maternal or familial concerns. Third, fetal life is to be protected in all but a few exceptional instances. Thus some people regard permissive law as injustice to the fetus; others see restrictive laws as injustice to the woman. As Daniel Callahan has noted:

The essence of the moral problem in abortion is the proper way in which to balance the rights of the unborn . . . against the right of a woman not to have a child she does not want.[58]

The evaluation of unborn life in the face of the competing interests of the woman is not only the heart of the moral problem; it is also the heart of the feasibility problem. If one thinks abortion is the wrongful killing of human life, then one will want this reflected in law. For the key function of the law is to protect the most basic of all goods, human life. If, however, one thinks that many abortions are, for whatever reason, morally justifiable, this person will resent a very prohibitive public policy.

Where there is no agreement on the underlying evaluation, feasibility is at stake. For law must rest on a sufficiently broad shared conviction or on a very fundamental moral or constitutional principle that people are reluctant to deny. Without these broad bases, attempts to legislate will be futile, whether the law be permissive or restrictive.

What do we do when we are faced with profound conflict, where there is not agreement on the basic underlying equation? Some have suggested that present policy is a reasonably adequate way of living with conflict (no one forces another to have an abortion; no one forces another to carry a pregnancy). However, that is a deceptively simple point of view. What represents a better way of living with conflict will depend to some extent on what one supports as the resolution of the conflict. For example, if I grant that the conflict makes prohibitive law impracticable, but I believe (as a *moral* position) that nascent life is human life deserving of protection and hope that others come to share this view, then I might think the Supreme Court's decision simply deepens the difficulty of arriving at a resolution since it allows free abortion in a way that further blunts our sensitivities to the sanctity of nascent life. Widespread abortion is, after all, self-perpetuating.

The feasibility test is particularly difficult in our society. Ideally, where we are concerned with the rights of others, especially the most basic right to life, morality should translate easily into law. But the easier the translation, the less necessary the law. In other words, if this represents the ideal, it supposes it. *That* we do not have because moral evaluations of the fetus differ. In the present situation, a totally permissive law would deepen doubt and confusion and further erode respect for life; a very prohibitive policy would have enormous social costs in terms of other values.

In present conditions, therefore, we are confronted with a choice of two legal evils. The underlying conditions for good legislation are lacking. When confronted with two mutually exclusive options, both of which represent evils, we should choose the lesser evil. However, which option one sees as the lesser evil depends on many factors, but especially on one's evaluation of fetal life. Here again we are at an impasse.

What is to be done? Any moral position, whether that of Vatican II or that of the Supreme Court, is going to be experienced as an imposition. When we do not have shared convictions about substantive outcomes we turn to procedures. Indeed, the Supreme Court, once it had admitted that it did not know when life begins, should have remanded the matter to the legislature. In this spirit, many believe that the matter should, for the present, be decided in the legislature, where all have a chance to share in the democratic process. I say "for the present" because conditions are such that any legal disposition of the question must be accompanied by hesitation and large doses of dissatisfaction. That means that it is the right and duty of conscientious citizens to continue to debate the matter, to attempt to persuade in the public forum. For without persuasion, there will never be a sufficiently broad consensus. And without that, there will be no peaceable policy.

The American Catholic bishops have angered, and in some instances divided, their militant grass-roots constituency in two ways. First, in their 1983 pastoral letter ("The Challenge of Peace: God's Promise and Our Response"), they have linked their position on nuclear weapons to abortion as different aspects of defending life. Some anti-abortionists believe this coupling will spell political disaster for the anti-abortion cause because many advocates of a nuclear freeze are likely to retain their pro-abortion position.

Second, the bishops have publicly supported the Hatch proposal, which many consider a compromise. Senator Orrin Hatch's proposal, as modified by Senator Thomas Eagleton, states that "a right to abortion is not secured by this Constitution." It would thus effectively open the way for prohibitive state legislation. It was soundly defeated in the Senate.

Whatever one's position may be, Catholics must learn to distinguish between universally binding moral principles and specific applications. The latter allow for diversity of opinion, as the bishops rightly insist in their nuclear pastoral. This is a fortiori true of specific political choices. To fail to make this distinction is to degrade teaching authority. That is why the case of Agnes Mary Mansour is so tragic. It never should have happened. Mansour is absolutely orthodox on abortion, but favored Medicaid payments for abortion in the present circumstances. While I disagree with that judgment, I agree with the editors of *America* when they write: "To find her position on this issue unacceptable is vastly different from declaring her unfit for office or for religious life or unorthodox in Catholic doctrine."[59]

Theologian Thomas E. Clarke, S.J., put the issue in its larger context as follows:

> Where then is the central issue in this sorry tale? The real questions, I believe, are those which touch the fidelity to the Gospel of certain church laws and procedures, and the integrity of their interpretation and application by churchmen within diverse cultural contexts. Does the new law of the church, for example, especially in its Roman interpretation, sufficiently respect the charismatic character of religious life, and hence its greater autonomy as compared with the clerical state? What has happened to subsidiarity when the name of the Roman pontiff must be so readily invoked in settling local incidents of this nature? Will efforts to heed signs of the times forever have to yield to hardened categories inherited from a dying or dead past? And, most centrally perhaps, how can we develop ecclesiastical processes for dealing with baptized Christians which do not degrade those who participate in them? I am optimistic enough to think that we can find good answers to such basic questions, but only if we bring ourselves to name and eliminate the real obstacles to their being addressed.[60]

Bishop Thomas J. Gumbleton summarized Clarke's concerns by referring to the Church's treatment of Mansour as a "clear injustice."[61] Interesting in this respect is a pastoral letter of Francis T. Hurley, of Anchorage; Robert L. Whelan, S.J., of Fairbanks; and Michael H. Kenny, of Juneau. It concerns Proposition 6 and the withdrawal of public funding for abortion in Alaska. The bishops invite their diocesans to reflect and pray about this matter and "come to a decision." They are careful not to dictate the decision.[62]

A whole host of other questions are connected with the evaluation of fetal life. Three stand out: amniocentesis, fetal experimentation, and in utero surgery on the fetus. All three are likely to contain controversial aspects. The denominator common to them all is the application of a value judgment about the sanctity and inviolability of nascent life in the face of new technology.

Amniocentesis

At Georgetown University Medical Center, there are about six-hundred fifty amniocentesis procedures performed annually. About ten of these will reveal problem pregnancies. Five of them will end in abortion (not performed at Georgetown). If abortion were not legally available, the vast majority of these procedures would not be performed. This indicates the close relationship of most amniocentesis procedures with the availability of abortion.

Clearly this raises a delicate question. Should amniocentesis be easily available in a medical complex whose institutional policy as Catholic rejects abortion for fetal defect, a rejection of the chief reason for doing the procedure? A negative response would argue that since abortion is morally wrong for fetal defect, amniocentesis is a form of cooperation in what is morally wrong. It provides the information and thereby the stimulus toward what is morally wrong. Thus Kevin O'Rourke and Benedict Ashley conclude:

> Granted that abortion is ethically unacceptable, the counselor should not recommend amniocentesis unless it is justified by the possibility of intrauterine therapy of some type proportionate to the risks—a possibility which at present is still largely theoretical.[63]

They add further:

> If the parents declare a firm intention to abort (should there be fetal defect), the counselor should not cooperate in any way with them.

Is there no other approach to this question? I believe there is. It would build on the following empirical assumptions: 1) amniocentesis is easily available elsewhere; 2) amniocentesis will continue to be provided whether a Catholic facility is involved or not; 3) other facilities have less or no problem with abortion for fetal defect; 4) a Catholic facility must not undermine the normative stance of the Church; 5) a Catholic facility, being opposed to abortion, will provide counseling and support for continuing the pregnancy. The conclusion based on these assumptions is that by providing amniocentesis as a regular service, the Catholic facility will potentially and probably be involved in a service that will save fetal lives that would otherwise be lost.

Technically, amniocentesis (where an indication of fetal defect is followed by abortion) is a form of cooperation in the wrongdoing of another. But this cooperation is material, remote, and unnecessary—conditions that make it easier to justify. Thus, what O'Rourke and Ashley have stated about genetic counseling could be said of amniocentesis.

> Is it permissible for a counselor to give information to parents whom the counselor only suspects may resort to abortion? In the present ethical climate this suspicion always exists, and it has deterred Catholic health care facilities from instituting genetic counseling centers. However, parents have a right to such information which has good as well as bad uses, and the counselor who supplies it cooperates only materially and remotely if the parents use it for a purpose which the counselor considers unethical. In our opinion Catholic health care facilities have a duty to provide such counseling in accordance with Christian moral standards, since otherwise parents will be forced to obtain information from centers where abortion will be an accepted and even encouraged solution.[84]

This very same reasoning would apply to amniocentesis. But cooperation in the procedure means that both the institution and individual practitioners must be *prepared to* and *actually implement* a policy of support for the problem pregnancy. If they do not, the very reason for their participation in amniocentesis on a large scale has disappeared. They are simply part of a system making abortion more likely.

What does it mean to say that individuals must be prepared to and actually implement a support-the-pregnancy policy? *Negatively* it means that they should not recommend or encourage abortion. *Positively* it suggests four things: that they should reveal in their manner and attitude respect even for handicapped nascent life, they should be knowledgable about services and supports for the handicapped, they should be medically up to date about possibilities of lessening or correcting handicapping conditions, and they should be supporters of programs that aid the handicapped.

Implementing a policy of support for problem pregnancies requires extraordinary prudence because it means achieving the proper balance between respect for the consciences of parents and protection of the fetus, between compassion and coercion.

In Utero Interventions

The Guidelines speak of "supporting" life in the womb. One of those possible supports is in utero surgery. While this is still a new technique, there is little doubt that the technology will advance rapidly.

There are many aspects to this procedure that have ethical dimensions: for instance, safety, cost, risk to the mother, risk to the fetus, locus of decision. At some point or other, these dimensions are all intertwined and it is difficult to consider such cases abstractly in terms of a single dimension.

Let us take the case of fetoscopic insertion of a prosthesis to relieve intracranial pressure in the hydrocephalic fetus and closure of neural tube defects. The fetal pathology here is severe. If one looks merely at the fetal anomaly, it would be easy to conclude that the more severe the anomaly, the more justifiable is the assumption of risk in an attempt to correct it. Suppose, on the one hand, that the risk of causing abortion by attempted therapy is 50 percent. On the other hand, suppose that there is a 50 percent chance of complete success. One could easily conclude that the risk is justified, given the crippling character of retardation.

But that is not the whole picture. The procedure is invasive of the mother, with some associated risks. For this and other reasons, it is generally accepted that the parents are in control of the decision. The parents are faced with three options: do nothing and allow the pregnancy to come to term, abort, or accept the in utero surgery with its possible risk of failure or associated spontaneous abortion.

From a Catholic moral point of view, the second option is no option. The first option (do nothing) would depend on the state of the art and the risks to mother and fetus. As a general statement—and that only—I would suggest that where effective treatment is available and the risks are acceptably low, treatment is the only morally defensible alternative. However, those who hold a different moral position on abortion would view the matter differently. Specifically, since abortion would be viewed as a legitimate moral option, they would demand a much lower degree of maternal risk and a much higher success rate before suggesting the in utero surgery. Once again we see the central place of abortion in factoring out the ethical dimensions of *other* interventions.

One thing is clear with the advent of in utero surgery: the situation is more ambiguous than before. Earlier the options appeared to be two: bear a malformed child or have an abortion. Now we have an option we never had to think about before, the treatment option. Those who opt for abortion will have to face the thought that they could have—perhaps quite easily—not only saved the child but brought it healthy into this world.

Fetal Experimentation

Is it compatible with respect for germinating life to conduct experiments on such life, and most sharply, nontherapeutic experiments (that is, research not designed to improve the health conditions of the research subject by prophylactic, diagnostic, or treatment methods)? Dr. Maurice J. Mahoney of Yale University conducted a literature survey at the request of the National Commission for the Protection of Human Subjects. The survey covered the years of 1969–1974 and turned up some 3000 citations. Only a very small percentage of these concerned nontherapeutic research. But the problem is likely to grow with the increasing sophistication of intra-uterine technology.

As philosophers and theologians discussed this matter in the early 1970s two positions emerged. One was proposed vigorously by Paul Ramsey. Ramsey argued that fetuses and very young children cannot consent to such procedures and that without their consent the procedures are invasive in violation of the covenants that exist between human persons. Therefore he excludes all nontherapeutic research on fetuses.[65]

I myself argued that the fetus and the child are members of the human community and may be expected to render minimal service to that community if there is not significant cost to themselves. In other words, the child or the fetus could not reasonably object to such research if it offered significant hope of benefit (unattainable in other ways) without discernible risk.[66]

After a careful study of the two positions, a task force of the John XXIII Medical-Moral Research and Education Center concluded:

> The authors of this study are persuaded that both secular and Christian ethical humanism can accept the position of McCormick. They feel it can be safely granted that proxy consent may be given for nontherapeutic research in cases where, in McCormick's words, "there is no discernible risk or undue discomfort."[67]

Needless to note, I am delighted with such support. More important, however, is the issue itself. And in that regard, I am convinced that, given the appropriate conditions and safeguards, fetal experimentation would combine traditional respect for fetal life with the new technological capacity of allowing that life to be of service to others as it matures. While this may not be a Catholic idea as such, it is consistent with traditional Catholic concerns.

THE NEWBORN

18. *The problem of the newborn with disabilities is one of the most anguishing and difficult that Catholic institutions face. What is appropriate treatment must be determined by a balance of the benefit and burden of the treatment for the newborn. Treatments should not be extended where they offer no reasonable hope of benefit, or when the benefit is so overwhelmed by the burden that it must be said to be minimal and dispensable. Medical and surgical corrective procedures which are readily performed for otherwise healthy children should not be denied to handicapped children, unless the physical or mental handicap is so devastating that the child would derive no benefit from correction. Whatever their condition, these infants should never be the subjects of nontherapeutic research which risks harming them in any significant way. Every possible effort should be made to offer them and their families love, affection, and tenderness during their short lives.*

Guideline 18 calls attention to the "anguishing and difficult" dimension of treatment decisions for the newborn. These decisions are anguishing because they are often life-or-death decisions, and are colored by profound emotions and loyalty bonds. They are difficult because they are often surrounded by doubts and uncertainties.

Both here and in Guideline 21, the language used is "appropriate treatment"—and, correlatively by implication, "inappropriate." This language was chosen to avoid the terms, *ordinary* and *extraordinary*. These terms have been used for some decades, first within the Catholic community, then by a much broader public, including the American Medical Association (1974). The AMA House of Delegates, after rejecting intentional (mercy) killing, continues:

> The cessation of the employment of extraordinary means to prolong the life of the body when there is irrefutable evidence that biological death is imminent is the decision of the patient and/or his immediate family.[68]

Traditionally, if a medical intervention had to be qualified as ordinary, it was seen as morally mandatory. If extraordinary, it was not morally mandatory. It was said to be ordinary if it offered a reasonable hope of benefit to the patient *and* could be used without excessive inconvenience (risk, pain, expense, etc.). If it offered no reasonable hope of benefit *or* was excessively burdensome, it was extraordinary.

Many people in the field (for example, Robert Veatch, Paul Ramsey, and James Childress) believe that this terminology has outlived its usefulness. There are several reasons for this. First, the terminology too easily hides the nature of the judgment being made. The major reference point in factoring out what is "reasonable" (benefit) and "excessive" (burden) is the patient—his or her condition, biography, prognosis, and values. The terminology, however, suggests that attention should fall on the means in an all too mechanical way. Second, many people misinterpret the terms to refer to "what physicians ordinarily do, what is customary." This is not what the term means. In their ethical sense, they encompass many more dimensions of the situation than merely "what physicians ordinarily do." Thus the terms have been badly used in our recent history, especially as the vehicle for involuntary homicide, and, at the other end, as mandates for the fruitless and aimless prolongation of dying.

Many suggestions for replacements have been made. For instance, Paul Ramsey continues to suggest a "medical indications policy" (to rate certain options as either medically indicated or not medically indicated). This obscures the fact that we are dealing with a *moral* judgment, not a scientific one. The Sacred Congregation for the Doctrine of the Faith tentatively suggests "proportionate" and "disproportionate" means. Still others opt for "reasonable, fitting" and "unreasonable, unfitting." Finally, some prefer simply "high technology" and "low technology" responses.

Whatever the terms, in its excellent "Declaration on Euthanasia" (1980) the Congregation concludes:

> It will be possible to make a correct judgment as to the means by studying the type of treatment to be used, its degree of complexity or risk, its cost and possibilities of using it, and comparing these elements with the result that can be expected, taking into account the state of the sick person and his or her physical and moral resources.[69]

In brief, two elements anchor our judgments in life-sustaining judgments: *burden* and *benefit*. This means that life-sustaining interventions are not morally obligatory—for handicapped infants or anyone else—if they are either gravely burdensome or useless. These are, of course, value judgments, not mathematical equations, and the evaluation can be a close call.

It is this that Guideline 18 sets forth. It compares healthy with handicapped children and insists that the handicapped must receive medical and surgical corrective procedures readily given otherwise healthy children "unless the physical or mental handicap is so great that the child would derive no benefit from the procedure."

Several things should be noted here. First, this last qualifier is an attempt to provide a corrective to the rather heavy-handed intervention of the federal government in such situations in the wake of the "Infant Doe" case. On April 15, 1982, "Infant Doe," a week-old Down's syndrome baby, died in Bloomington, Indiana. The parents had obtained a court order barring doctors from feeding or treating him. The infant suffered from tracheo-esophageal fistula, a condition that, unless surgically corrected, prevents ingestion of food. This case received widespread publicity and aroused a great deal of public concern about the protection of newborn infants. Indeed, Richard S. Schweiker, Secretary of the Department of Health and Human Services, stated on May 18, 1982, that "the president has instructed me to make absolutely clear to health care providers in this nation that federal law does not allow medical discrimination against handicapped infants." At the same time, Betty Lou Dotson, director of HHS's Office for Civil Rights, sent a letter to the nation's nearly seven thousand hospitals reminding them of the applicability of section 504 of the Rehabilitation Act (1973) to these cases. That section stipulates:

> No otherwise qualified handicapped individual . . . shall, solely by reason of his handicap, be excluded from the participation in, be denied the benefits of, or be subjected to discrimination under any program or activity receiving federal financial assistance.[70]

Dotson's letter to the hospitals stated:

> Under section 504 it is unlawful for a recipient of federal financial assistance to withhold from a handicapped infant nutritional sustenance or medical or surgical treatment required to correct a life-threatening condition if: 1) the withholding is based on the fact that the infant is handicapped; and 2) the handicap does not render the treatment or nutritional sustenance medically contraindicated.

One of the grave problems with such an approach is the imprecision of the term *handicap*. After all, the reason we do not bring lifesaving treatment to some patients is precisely that their handicap is so severe (for example, metastatic carcinoma) that prolongation of life is no longer in their best interest. Clearly then, as Norman Frost, M.D., notes, "handicap . . . is a morally valid reason for withholding treatment *in some* cases."[71] It is this imprecision that Guideline 18 seeks to correct.

The correction is, however, general in character. It states simply, "would derive no benefit from correction." What instances fall within this category? Can more concrete guidelines be provided? Perhaps not. But hesitantly I have suggested possible specifications for this most difficult problem. Perhaps the burden-benefit evaluation could be clarified by the following four points.

First, lifesaving interventions ought not be omitted for institutional or managerial reasons. Included in this specification is the ability of this particular family to cope with a badly disabled baby. This idea is likely to be controversial because there are many who believe that the child is the ultimate victim when parents unsuited to the challenge of a disadvantaged baby must undertake the task. Still, it remains an unacceptable erosion of our respect for life to make the gift of life once given depend on the personalities and emotional or financial capacities of the parents alone. No one ought to be allowed to die simply because the parents are not up to the task. At this point society has certain responsibilities. To face these agonizing situations by allowing the child to die will merely blunt society's sensitivities to its unfulfilled social responsibilities.

Second, life-sustaining interventions may not be omitted simply because the baby is retarded. There may be further complications associated with retardation that justify withholding life-sustaining treatment. But retardation alone, as both Chief Justice Givan of the Indiana Supreme Court and Lord Justice Templeman of the British court of appeals made clear, is not an indication for nontreatment. To claim otherwise is a slur on the condition of the retarded, one that would mandate fundamentally unequal treatment of equals.

Third, life-sustaining intervention may be omitted or withdrawn when it imposes excessive hardship on the patient, especially when this combines with poor prognosis (for example, repeated cardiac surgery, low-prognosis transplants, increasingly iatrogenic oxygenization for low-birthweight babies).

Fourth, life-sustaining interventions may be omitted or withdrawn at a point when it becomes clear that life can be prolonged only for a relatively brief time and only with the continued use of artificial feeding (as, for example, in some cases of necrotizing enterocolitis).

These norms, I believe, provide some guidance for the types of cases under discussion. Here the phrase "some guidance" must be emphasized. Concrete rules such as these do not mandate decisions. They neither replace prudence nor eliminate conflicts and doubts. They are simply attempts to provide outlines of the areas in which prudence should operate. They do not replace parental-physician responsibility, but are an attempt to enlighten it. If even good and loving parents can make mistakes—and they can and have—then there ought to be some criteria (even if general) by which we can judge the decision to be right or wrong, for ethical persons ought to be reason-giving persons.

However, doubts and agonizing problems will remain. Hence a certain range of choices must be allowed to parents, a certain margin of error, a certain space. Guidelines can be developed to help us to judge when parents have exceeded the limits of human discretion. Guidelines cannot cover every instance where human discretion must intervene. The margin of error tolerable should reflect not only the utter finality of the decision (which tends to narrow it) but also the unavoidable uncertainty and doubt (which tends to broaden it).

Another point to note about Guideline 18 is that it is the precipitate of a general value judgment on the meaning of life and death: it is this value judgment that must constantly be adapted to new medical circumstances. This is another way of saying "tradition in transition." In the past the Catholic tradition has attempted to walk a balanced middle path between medical vitalism (that preserves life at any cost) and medical pessimism (that kills when life seems frustrating, burdensome, and useless). Both of these extremes are rooted in an identical idolatry of life—an attitude that, at least by inference, views death as an unmitigated, absolute evil, and life as the absolute good. The middle course that has structured Catholic attitudes is that life is indeed a basic and precious good, but a good to be preserved precisely as the condition of other values. As the Sacred Congregation for the Doctrine of the Faith worded it in 1980: "Human life is the basis of all goods, and is the necessary source and condition of every human activity and of all society."[72] It is these other values and possibilities that underlie the duty to preserve physical life and that also dictate the limits of this duty. In other words, life is a relative good, and the duty to preserve it is a limited one. The Catholic tradition maintains that there are values more important than life in the living of life. So, it also holds that there are values more important than life in dying. For this reason, the accumulation of minutes of life is not the moral guideline by which dying must be done. For instance, the justification for administering pain-killing drugs, *even if they shorten life*, recognizes that there is a value in being pain-free that permits the pursuit of other values, such as prayer.

Where does this value judgment on the meaning of life and death originate? From the Christian story, as indicated above. That story tells us the ultimate meaning for ourselves and the world. It tells us the kind of people we ought to be, the goods we ought to pursue, the dangers we ought to avoid, the kind of world we ought to seek. As Vatican II put it: "Faith throws a new light on everything, manifests God's design for man's total vocation, and thus directs the mind to solutions which are fully human." In this "design" we are, after Jesus' example, pilgrims with no lasting home here. We are offered, in and through Jesus, eternal life. Our greatest achievement is genuine love for each other. And "there is no greater love than this: to lay down one's life for one's friends" (John 15:13). In these perspectives death is not an unconditioned evil nor is life as we know it an absolute good.

THE RETARDED

The United Nations proclaimed 1981 the International Year of Disabled Persons. In conjunction with this the Holy See published its "Document of the Holy See for the International Year of Disabled Persons."[73] After calling attention to the unrepeatable value of the individual person and the inviolability of her or his rights, the statement insists that the basic principles for dealing with the disabled are the principles of integration, normalization, and personalization.

The principle of integration "opposes the tendency to isolate, segregate, and neglect the disabled." It includes more positively a commitment to make the disabled person "a subject in the fullest sense." The principle of normalization involves an effort to ensure the complete rehabilitation of the disabled person by providing an environment as close as possible to the normal. The principle of personalization emphasizes the fact that in the various forms of treatment, "it is always the dignity, welfare, and total development of the handicapped person, in all his or her dimensions and physical, moral, and spiritual faculties that must be primarily considered, protected, and promoted." Upon these three principles the document builds very helpful concrete suggestions about dealing with the handicapped, especially the retarded.

Over a two-year period I had the privilege of working with a group of Catholic laypeople, nuns, and priests involved in the apostolate to the retarded. Our conversations led to the development of a set of practical guidelines that could be of help to those involved in this apostolate. While all the conversation partners contributed valuable additions, I accept full responsibility for them in their present form: they are reproduced here as a concrete instance of "Catholic consciousness" responding to the condition of mental retardation, and therefore as an instance of tradition in transition. A few explanatory comments will be added at the end.

"ETHICAL GUIDELINES FOR THE TREATMENT OF THE MENTALLY RETARDED"

Introduction

As Catholic people of faith, we welcome all human life as a gift from God, the Creator and Redeemer. As loving people, we share life with one another and hold ourselves responsible to support and nourish life. As a hopeful people, we are called to search together for general orientations, guidelines, and reference points to help us confront concrete life situations that require human prudence, discernment, and courage. We reject the notion that all kinds of mental and physical impairment are consequences of sin and manifestations of evil. Yet we admit the limits of our understanding of some of the suffering that accompanies these disabilities. Our faith in God's good purpose is not thereby diminished. Our goal is to build a network of support among us through which decisions can be made in faithful response to a loving God. Persons who are mentally retarded are both God's gift and challenge. These principles and guidelines are an attempt to acknowledge this gift and respond to this challenge in our times.

Principles from Which the Guidelines Follow

1. Persons with the conditions of mental retardation are persons equal in dignity to all other human beings. Therefore, in what concerns their rights, privileges and responsibilites, the same guidelines and principles which apply to society as a whole should apply to them as far as possible.
2. Moral decisions affecting retarded persons should be their own. Or, they should be educated, supported, and encouraged to participate in the decisionmaking process as far as possible.
3. The basic moral criterion for decisions relating to retarded persons should be the same as for other persons, whether they can make their own decisions or not; that is to say, his/her overall good within the framework of the common good consistent with the rights and privileges stated in Number 1.

4. In our Catholic Christian perspective the good of the whole person involves spiritual, intellectual, physical, emotional, and social development.
    a) The spiritual development of the person means access to the full richness of Christian traditions (religious education, sacraments, community life).
    b) The intellectual development involves adequate educational opportunities.
    c) The physical development includes physical integrity, health and growth, and adequate health care.
    d) Emotional and social development involves opportunities for affirming their own self-worth, for friendships and for other forms of affective relationships.
5. Pastoral judgments about the appropriate combinations of these areas of development in the individual case must consider the person's entire framework of life.
6. In responding to the behavior and development of retarded persons, as well as any other persons, several important distinctions must always be kept in mind:
    a) the difference between the ideally possible and the practical capacity
    b) the difference between impulsive conduct and premeditated conduct
    c) the difference between morally wrong conduct and annoying conduct.
7. Like anyone else, retarded persons share in the fallen but redeemed condition of human nature. Therefore, the standard impediments to freedom (namely, habit, force, fear, and passion) should be considered with special sensitivity to the condition of the mentally retarded person.
8. One of the unnecessary sufferings of retarded persons is the attitude of the general population. The inherent value and dignity of retarded persons does not come from the fact that they are retarded, but from the very fact of their own personhood and humanity. This means two things: first, we must align our attitudes personally and socially to respond to them as persons with their handicap but not exclusively through it; second, we must do all that is morally possible to alleviate, correct, and prevent the handicapping condition, and to facilitate their reaching a full potential.
9. In some situations the moral dilemma is present in which only nega-

tive options appear available (protective sterilization vs. protective custody, as an example). In such situations the option should be chosen that is least damaging to the individual and any others involved, and that attempts to realize all the values possible for the individual.

Moral Guidelines

Moral Education

1. Since retarded persons have both rights and responsibilities, they have the right to a truly moral education which will prepare them for the proper acceptance and exercise of these rights and responsibilities.
2. Such an education is one which gradually opens them to and motivates them toward the positive values of truth, honesty, self-discipline. Moral education cannot be identified with institutional control, mere public propriety awareness, mere punishment-reward stimuli.
3. To achieve such gradual growth and motivation, responsibility for decisions should be increasingly entrusted to the individual wherever possible, with appropriate accounting and follow-up.
4. Proper moral education must include education of peers, parents, and guardians of the retarded person to expect appropriate responsibility and not mere conformity from the retarded person.
5. Where certain forms of training and behavior adjustment, as an aspect of early moral education, are concerned, it must be noted that such techniques can touch the basic freedom of acting on one's own behalf. Therefore, they should be used not simply to facilitate management, though that may be a factor, but with the person's overall good in mind. Toward this end, both behavior and modification techniques need careful evaluation by responsible personnel prior to and during use of these techniques.

Sexuality and Affectivity

1. The total well-being of the retarded person includes affective and sexual components. These ought to be met in a positive way in accordance with the age and capacity of the individual.
2. The overall guiding principle in meeting these needs is the long-term welfare, adjustment and health of the individual. Such a principle cannot be replaced by primary consideration of institutional convenience and efficiency. Nor can such a principle be applied in an automatic or mechanistic way.

3. Proper education to and provision for the affective and sexual needs of the individual should avoid the enticing to sexual activity he/she cannot understand or handle in a constructive way. It must also avoid undue social isolation and constraints.

4. This means that sound education will provide increasing insight into the meaning of sexuality and viable alternatives to sexual acting out, that is, other constructive outlets for sexual energy and desire. While sexual intimacy ought to be restricted to marriage, still it is understandable that special problems can arise. However, it must be remembered that heterosexual friendships are a positive part of a person's normal growth. The development and direction of such friendships should be treated on an individual basis.

5. Masturbation should be viewed and approached neither moralistically nor punitively, but realistically as a normal growth phenomenon—perhaps over a very long period of time—requiring understanding and patience, but not overemphasis.

6. Homosexual inclinations as well as overt activity should be approached with great compassion and understanding. They should be viewed as an opportunity for and challenge to individual counseling and perhaps growth beyond such sexual expression.

7. Moral rape (i.e., involuntary intercourse) refers to situations where the person does not sufficiently understand the meaning and implications of what is occurring and therefore cannot be judged to be giving sufficiently free consent. The following considerations must be weighed to determine whether acts of physical intimacy constitute moral rape in an individual case:
   a) the person's understanding of the meaning of sexual intercourse
   b) the person's ability to enter into positive and constructive interpersonal relationships
   c) the person's ability to perceive what is right and wrong in personal behavior
   d) the person's ability to act upon moral perceptions of rightfulness and wrongfulness.

8. To insure that protective measures against moral rape are truly *that*, and in the person's best interest, such measures must be reevaluated on an ongoing basis.

9. Contraceptive agents may be used as protection against pregnancy when it is judged that likely sexual relations, which cannot be humanely prevented, would fall into the category of moral rape. Sterilizing interventions in similar circumstances must be viewed as last resorts and

154: Health and Medicine in the Catholic Tradition

as such should be relatively rare occurrences. If they are justifiable in
individual cases, this can be concluded only after the parents or guardians (if there are such) have been consulted and state or Federal stat-
utes have been fully observed.
10. If pregnancy occurs, it should be supported as fully as possible in conformity with a basic respect for life.

Marriage
1. While there are several lifestyles that ought to be made available and
presented to retarded persons, nonetheless the right to marry and benefit from the graces of the sacrament is a basic right. It must be presumed to be present until incapacity is clear. In other words, it is the
severity of mental retardation and not the condition as such which
may constitute a barrier to marriage.
2. In assessing the capacity to marry and advisability of marriage, the
following qualities of the couple should be considered by them and by
those assisting them to make their decisions: their consistency and
commitment, their emotional maturity to solve problems, their level
of social awareness, their freedom to decide to marry, their respect
and devotion to each other, and their autonomy in ordinary living.
Furthermore, the capacity to marry should not be identified with the
capacity to rear children.
3. Since both marriage and childbearing involve grave challenges and
burdens, sometimes beyond the isolated capacities of the individuals,
the retarded persons need and deserve *special* practical supports of
family, friends, and church in this undertaking.
4. Preparation for marriage, while adapted to the special needs of retarded persons, should be no less thorough for them than for other persons and should take on the perspectives of their total life style. It should
include not only education in sexuality, the advisability of childbearing (including genetic counseling when deemed advisable), and the
practical tasks of childbearing and childrearing, but also in communication, economics, and home management.

Medical Treatment
1. The "Ethical and Religious Directives for Catholic Health Facilities"
provide helpful guidelines for the medical treatment of the retarded
person. However, because of diminished mental capacity and, in some
cases, the institutionalized condition of the person, special attention
needs to be given to the following directives:

a) (no. 3) Any patient, regardless of the extent of his/her physical or psychic disability, has a right to be treated with respect consonant with his/her dignity as a person.

b) (no. 5) Any procedure potentially harmful to the patient is morally justified only insofar as it is designed to produce a proportionate good for the patient.

c) (no. 6) Ordinarily the proportionate good that justifies a medical or surgical procedure should be the total good of the patient himself/herself. ("Ordinarly," consult 4 below.)

d) (no. 9) The duties of professional secrecy must be carefully fulfilled (sc., charts and records, as well as regards confidential matters learned in the exercise of professional duties).

e) Adequate spiritual care must be available to the sick (retarded) person. This refers to spiritual counseling, easy availability of the sacraments, and appropriate preparation for one's own death and the death of others, and the expectation of a full Christian burial.

2. "The respect consonant with the dignity of the person" demands that wherever possible informed consent of the patient must be obtained for medical procedures. In some instances, this may be realistically impossible; in such cases assent (nonobjection of the patient) may suffice together with the consent of the legal authorized representative of the individual; or even parent or guardian consent may (in very severe instances) be sufficient.

3. Research procedures which present the possibility of direct benefit to the individual subject and
   a) which involve *minimal risks only* may be undertaken subject to the consent of the guidelines above
   b) which involve *more than minimal risks* may be undertaken subject to the consent of the guidelines above and if
      • the risk is justified by the prospect of benefit to the subject
      • the relation of risk to anticipated benefit is at least as favorable as that presented by available alternative approaches.

4. Research procedures which present no possibility of direct benefit to the individual subject shall never be done when alternate populations are available. When alternate populations are not available those procedures which
   a) involve *minimal risk only* may be undertaken subject to the consent requirements stated above and approval of an Institutional Review Board;

    b) involve *more than minimal risk* may not be undertaken unless
- the risk presents a minor increase over minimal risk
- the anticipated knowledge is of vital importance for the understanding or amelioration of the type of disorder or condition of the subject, or may be reasonably expected to benefit the subject in the future
- consent requirements as stated above are observed
- an Institutional Review Board has approved the procedure.

5. No treatment, whether palliative, corrective, or life-preserving, should be withheld or terminated simply because a person is retarded.

Under "Sexuality and Affectivity" (above) item 9 states that agents, including as a last resort sterilization, are allowed for protection against "moral rape." Perhaps it was item 9 that led the episcopal moderator of the apostolate to the retarded to reject for publication the directives formulated by the apostolate to the retarded. Whatever the case, it must be recalled that in 1961 three prominent Roman theologians concluded that sterilization was permissible as self-protection against the threat of rape in certain cases. The theologians were P. Palazzini, F. Hürth, S.J., and F. Lambruschini.[74] They considered sterilizing interventions in such coercive circumstances to fall outside the Church's condemnation of sterilization. Item 9 adopts a similar position—and thus it does not touch at all on the official (for example, *Humanae vitae*) condemnation of sterilization.

Under "Marriage" (above) item 2 distinguishes the capacity to marry from the capacity to rear children. To some this may appear to involve an invalidating intention against children. It does not. Pius XII stated about the duty to procreate:

> Serious motives, such as those which are frequently present in the so-called "indications"—medical, eugenic, economic, and social—can exempt from this positive, obligatory duty for a long time, *even for the entire duration of the marriage.*[75]

THE AGED

19. *Health care providers should respect the continuing right of older persons to bear primary responsibility for decisions regarding their care. Providers should also recognize and respond to the special issues related to the care of the older person, e.g., privacy, sexuality, grieving, interaction of diseases; and coping with loss, progressive limitation, and depression.*

This Guideline singles out a particularly vulnerable population, the aged. Often the aging process entails a diminution of physical and mental powers and a growing dependency on others. In the health care setting this too often translates into a passivity that invites manipulation and paternalism. Against this background the Guideline asserts the continuing autonomy of the older person as a part of his or her basic dignity.

It then refers to "special issues" in the care of the elderly. Throughout the United States, I have heard nurses complain about the hospital treatment of the elderly. "It is just plain sad," one said recently. "They cannot defend themselves or retaliate, and often enough cannot make their needs clear. They are sitting ducks for insensitive personnel and for an impersonal health care system."

All of us, of course, suffer under faceless impersonality. But the elderly are especially vulnerable because of their dependency and loneliness. There are three factors at work that intensify this problem. First, there is the awesome growth of technology. Everything from diagnosis to acute care to billing is done by computer. Check the advertisements in any medical journal and it becomes clear that medicine and the machine are wed. This gives efficiency, but also impersonality.

Second, there is cost and cost containment. Spiraling costs are due to many factors (for example, sophistication of services, higher wages, more personnel, cost pass-along systems, and inflation). In 1976, for example, expenditures for health constituted 11.4 percent of the national budget. Of this sum, 91 percent went into health care systems, 3 percent to human biology, 5 percent to environmental factors, and 1 percent to lifestyle. Obviously, the cost factor will present difficult decisions. Shall we rescind federal coverage of end-stage renal disease? In England, few over fifty-five get government-paid dialysis. That contains a message for the elderly.

Another factor is the multiplication of what I call "public entities" in health care delivery. I mean attorneys, courts, and legislatures. We have legislated living wills: we have *Quinlan, Saikewicz, Fox, Spring, Storar, Perlmutter.* We have the *Wade, Bolton* decisions (1973) of the Supreme Court. These are but the tip of the iceberg.

Together these factors affect the very matrix of the healing profession. This matrix roots in the conviction that patient-management decisions must be tailor-made to the individual, to the individual's condition and values. They are *personal* decisions that must suit the individual. Yet the three factors mentioned above are rather *impersonal* factors. When they begin to preprogram our treatment, they tend to depersonalize that treatment. The impact on the elderly can be especially devastating. Adverting to this problem may be half of its solution, just as inadvertence will only compound it.

The growing depersonalization of health care can be a great threat to the elderly, who need time, touching, and tenderness. But this threat is powerfully supported by a cluster of cultural attitudes. Victorina Peralta, director of adult and aging services for the Philadelphia Department of Public Welfare, highlights the following qualities of our culture: youth-oriented, production-oriented, pill-oriented, speed-oriented, highly mobile, success-oriented, waste-oriented, "latest-model" oriented, work-oriented, dollar-oriented, cosmetic-oriented, swinging, having versus being, strength-oriented.[76]

Perhaps the most prominient quality of the lives of the elderly is dependence. For this reason Drew Christiansen, S.J., develops what he calls a "theology of dependence."[77] For most of our adult lives (except for grave ill-nesses or major setbacks) we can and do ignore the dependence that ties us to other men and women. As Christiansen puts it:

> We keep the realization of our need for others at arm's length by keeping busy. If we can produce enough, if we can win enough, if we can party enough, we don't have to think too long about the meaning of life. More-over, by manipulating things and managing people, we convince our-selves of our freedom and mastery of the world, and so avoid admitting how much we owe to others and to God.[78]

Christiansen sees this avoidance of dependence as mistaken. Dependence is an opportunity, a call to let ourselves go, to open up to God, to cling in trust to a power beyond our control, to see more clearly than ever the source and end of life. But if the elderly are to view their own aging in this way, it must be through the mediating kindness of others. Christiansen continues:

> The responsibilities of the family, friends, and associates of the enfeebled elderly, therefore, are awesome, for it falls on them to restore the trust of their aged companions in life and in the Author of life. Dependent aging, if you will, is a sacrament of life, and relatives and friends are its ministers.

Interestingly enough, this "ministering" to the dependent elderly should expand their autonomy at this time of diminishing personal powers. In the kindness of others they are allowed to glimpse the kindness of the good God. Dependence on others should be a sign of our more radical dependence on God. Since our freedom is intended to lead us to a deeper union with God, it is an interesting paradox that our deep dependence on God establishes our own radical independence: independence in dependence!

Thus from a theological perspective, dependent old age should represent a flowering rather than a wilting. Or, as Christiansen nicely words it:

> Outside of faith, dependence threatens us with subjugation, and our self-assertion may lead to isolation and abandonment. But for those who believe in the Giver of life, the promise hidden in dependence is communion with the Source of life itself.[79]

Teilhard de Chardin composed a prayer that summarizes this beautifully. In part, it goes as follows:

> Now that I have found the joy of utilizing all forms of growth to make you, or to let you, grow in me, grant that I may willingly consent to this last phase of communion in the course of which I shall possess you by diminishing in you.
>
> When the signs of age begin to mark my body (and still more when they touch my mind); when the ill that is to diminish me or carry me off strikes from without or is born within me; when the painful moment comes in which I suddenly awaken to the fact that I am ill or growing old; and above all that last moment when I feel I am losing hold of myself and am absolutely passive within the hands of the great unknown forces that have formed me; in all those dark moments, O God, grant that I may understand that it is you (provided only my faith is strong enough) who are painfully parting the fibers of my being in order to penetrate to the very marrow of my substance and bear me away within yourself.[80]

Such a theology should be the prism through which a Catholic views the aging process. In this sense Guideline 19 and its reference to "the continuing right of older persons to bear primary responsibility for decisions regarding their care" opens up and stems from a theological understanding of life. If health care providers share that understanding, they will be much more likely to "respect the continuing right of older persons." For they will view older persons in an entirely different way—as persons expanding their independence through dependence.

Conclusion

A transition involves both a "coming from" and a "going toward." The former dimension refers to a past that is historical but neither dead nor to be sloughed off like a decaying shell. This past was alive, with its own enduring visions, motives, and values that must continue to animate the "going toward" in ever changing circumstances. Catholic health care is in a state of transition, as it ought to be. A symptom of this transition is chapter 4, on justice: it is the shortest chapter in this book; in five years it will, or should be, the longest chapter in any discussion of Catholic health care.

An attempt to detail precisely the characteristics of this transition would be presumptuous. But no prophetic gift is required to point out several emerging emphases. First, there must and will be more collegiality in the establishment of policy for health care institutions. The remarkable pastoral letter of the American Catholic bishops, "The Challenge of Peace," points unmistakably in this direction. If there are no simple answers to complex problems in the sphere of peace and war, the same must be said of health care. To face the challenges of the future, sensitivity to scientific data, local variations, and many competences is an absolute must. This will require consultation and collegiality.

Second (and this emphasis is closely connected with the first), things will tend to remain in transition. Very few things can be carved in stone given the rapid changes that are occurring in health care in general. This suggests that Catholic health care facilities must develop a kind of tolerance for the tentative.

Third, one can detect in the transitional phase a growing rejection of individualism in health care and the emergence of a communal consciousness. Catholic tradition, with its emphasis on the person as a social being, should be well-prepared for this adjustment.

Finally, I detect a shift from ethical limitations to a more aggressive attitude of pursuit. There is an emerging awareness of the global character of health care and a corresponding focus on the positive responsibility for provision of health care.

What concrete form these emphases will take in the future is difficult to say. One thing seems certain: transition is usually not without a kind of last-gasp neurological twitch that reveals the pain of the transition. But this should be expected in a pilgrim Church that exists in diverse cultures and rapidly changing times—to say nothing of existing "between the times." Furthermore, it should be welcomed with hope and joy by a Church at whose center stands the crucified, but risen and glorified, Christ. For ever since Christ, death and resurrection have been the paradigm of tradition in transition.

Notes

Introduction

1. Eugene Kennedy, "The End of the Immigrant Church," *Illinois Issues* (August 1982): 15–21.
2. Joseph Cardinal Bernardin, *Loyola Magazine* (Summer 1983): 3.
3. John Howard Yoder, "The Hermeneutics of Peoplehood: A Protestant Perspective on Practical Moral Reasoning." *Journal of Religious Ethics* 10 (1982): 40–67.
4. *Documents of Vatican II*, ed. Walter Abbott, S.J. (New York: America, 1966), p. 715. Hereafter, *Documents*.
5. *Documents*, p. 715.

Chapter 2/Well-Being

1. Pius XII, "Allocution to the First International Congress of Histopathology," in *The Human Body: Papal Teachings*, selected and arranged by the Monks of Solesmes (Boston: St. Paul Editions, 1960), nn. 349–81; *Acta Apostolicae Sedis* 44 (1952): 779–89.
2. *Documents*, p. 256.
3. *Schema constitutionis pastoralis de Ecclesia in mundo huius temporis: Expensio modorum partis secundae* (Rome: Typ. pol. Vat., 1965), pp. 37–38.
4. Louis Janssens, "Artificial Insemination: Ethical Considerations," *Louvain Studies* 8 (1980): 3–29.
5. *Summa Theologica* I–II, q. 91, a. 2.
6. Janssens, op. cit., p. 11.
7. Cited in Janssens, p. 11.
8. *Documents*, p. 201.
9. *Documents*, p. 211.
10. *Documents*, p. 267.
11. *Documents*, p. 271.
12. *Documents*, p. 273.
13. F. Hürth, S.J., "La fécondation artificielle. Sa valeur morale et juridique," *Nouvelle revue théologique* 68 (1946): 413.

14. Ibid., p. 415.
15. Ibid., p. 416.
16. Thomas E. Clarke, S.J., "Touching in Power: Our Health System," in *Above Every Name: The Lordship of Christ and Social Systems* (Ramsey, NJ: Paulist, 1980), p. 253.
17. Ibid., p. 253.
18. Ibid., p. 259.
19. Walter J. Burghardt, S.J., "The Health Apostolate: Service, Understanding, Wonder," *Hospital Progress* 64 (February 1983): 30–36.
20. Joseph H. Fichter, S.J., *Religion and Pain* (New York: Crossroad, 1981).
21. Ibid., p. 108.
22. William Kenney and Charles Ceronsky, "Developing Christian Values in a Catholic Health Facility," *Hospital Progress* 55 (October 1974): 32.
23. *Catholic Chronicle*, 25 Feb. 1983.
24. Lawrence K. Altman, "Hospital Patients Can Suffer Twice When Staff Adds Insult to Injuries," *New York Times*, 22 Feb. 1983, sec. C.
25. *Catholic Chronicle*, 25 Feb. 1983.
26. Quentin Quesnell, *The Gospel of Christian Freedom* (New York: Herder and Herder, 1969), p. 63.
27. Luke 22.
28. Mark 10.
29. Harris Wofford, *Of Kennedys and Kings: Making Sense of the Sixties* (New York: Farrar-Straus-Giroux, 1980), p. 281.
30. Johannes B. Metz, *Followers of Christ* (Ramsey, NJ: Paulist, 1978), pp. 39–40.
31. William F. May, *A Catalogue of Sins* (New York: Holt, Rinehart and Winston, 1967), p. 50.
32. Joseph Sittler, *The Structure of Christian Ethics* (New Orleans: Louisiana State University Press, 1958), p. 25.
33. Ibid., p. 45.
34. John 1:3.
35. Walter Kasper, *An Introduction to Christian Faith* (Ramsey, NJ: Paulist, 1980), p. 82.
36. Sittler, op. cit., p. 46.
37. Ibid., p. 25.
38. Ibid., p. 11.
39. Enrico Chiavacci, "The Grounding for the Moral Norm in Contemporary Theological Reflection," in *Readings in Moral Theology*, vol. 2 (Ramsey, NJ: Paulist, 1980), pp. 291–92.
40. Ibid., p. 288.
41. Sittler, op. cit., p. 18.
42. Ibid., p. 33.
43. Chiavacci, op. cit., p. 288.
44. Ibid., p. 288.
45. Sittler, op. cit., p. 36.
46. Ibid., pp. 50–51.
47. Romans 13:10.
48. 1 John 4:8, 16.

49. 1 John 4:10.
50. Romans 5:8; Matthew 5:45.
51. John 1:49.
52. John 15:13.
53. John 15:10.
54. Romans 12: 4–5.
55. Ephesians 4:13–15.
56. Galatians 2:20.
57. Luke 9:23.
58. John 4:14, 14:21.
59. John 13:33–35.
60. John 15:12–13.
61. Matthew 22:37–38.
62. Romans 13:8–9; Galatians 5:14.
63. 1 Corinthians 13:1–3.
64. Ephesians 3–17.
65. Colossians 3:12–14.
66. John 13:34.
67. 2 Corinthians 5:17.
68. John 13:35.
69. John 17:20–23.
70. L. Cerfaux, O.P., "La Charité fraternelle et le retour du Christ," *Ephémerides Theologicae Lovanienses* 24 (1958): 326.
71. Cf. G. Gilleman, S.J., *The Primacy of Charity in Moral Theology* (Westminster, Md.: Newman Press, 1959).
72. Cf. note 71.
73. Cf. note 31.
74. May, op. cit., p. 28.
75. Ibid., p. 33.
76. Ibid., p. 35.
77. John 13:34.
78. Raymond Brown, S.S., *The Gospel According to John* (Garden City, NJ: Doubleday, 1970), p. 612.
79. It is not clear to me how we can love one another *as* Jesus did in the first sense, so as "to bring about their salvation," unless it is that our loving faith is a channel for *his* love (saving grace) to others.
80. Cf. *The Spiritual Exercises of St. Ignatius*, ed. Louis J. Puhl, S.J. (Westminster, Md.: Newman Press, 1953), p. 69.
81. Metz, op. cit., p. 40.
82. Sittler, op. cit., p. 69.
83. Cf. *Documents*, pp. 489–521. An apostolate is here defined as all activity that brings "all persons to share in Christ's saving redemption and that through them the whole world might in actual fact be brought into fellowship with him," p. 491.
84. Sittler, op. cit., p. 64.
85. *Documents*, p. 498.
86. *Documents*, p. 499.

87. May, op. cit., p. 63.
88. *Documents*, p. 493.
89. Ibid.
90. *Documents*, p. 505.
91. Thomas Clarke, S.J., *Above Every Name* (Ramsey, NJ: Paulist, 1980), p. 252.
92. *Documents*, p. 493.
93. From an unpublished manuscript.
94. Albert R. Jonsen, Mark Siegler, and William J. Winslade, *Clinical Ethics* (New York: Macmillan, 1982).
95. Sittler, op. cit., p. 64.

Chapter 3/Morality

1. This and the citations in the following two paragraphs are from *Doing Evil to Achieve Good*, ed. Paul Ramsey and Richard A. McCormick, S.J. (Chicago: Loyola University Press, 1978), p. 194.
2. Yves Congar, O.P., "A Brief History of the Forms of the Magisterium," in *Readings in Moral Theology* vol. 3, ed. Charles E. Curran and Richard A. McCormick, S.J. (Ramsey, NJ: Paulist, 1982) p. 325.
3. *Documents*, p. 209.
4. *Documents*, p. 240.
5. *The Pope Speaks* 4 (1957) 45.
6. "Declaration on Euthanasia" (Vatican City: Vatican Polyglot Press, 1980); also *Origins* 10 (1980):154–57.
7. Franz Böckle, "Glaube und Handeln," in *Concilium* 120 (1976): 641–47.
8. "Declaration on Euthanasia," op. cit., 4.
9. Paul Ramsey, "Two-Step Fantastic: The Continuing Case of Brother Fox," *Theological Studies* 42 (1981): 122–34.
10. Daniel Callahan, "Shattuck Lecture: Contemporary Biomedical Ethics," *New England Journal of Medicine* 302, (May 29, 1980): 1232.
11. Ibid., p. 1233.
12. Cf. note 6.
13. Pius XII, *Acta Apostolicae Sedis* 49 (1957): 1031–32.
14. Paul Ramsey, "Liturgy and Ethics," *Journal of Religious Ethics* 7 (1979): 139–71.
15. Ibid.
16. Albert C. Outler, "The Beginning of Personhood: Theological Considerations," *Perkins Journal* 27 (1973): 28–34.
17. Ramsey, "Liturgy and Ethics," op. cit., p. 161.
18. James M. Gustafson, *The Contribution of Theology to Medical Ethics* (Milwaukee: Marquette, 1975), pp. 85–86.
19. Karl Rahner, *Theological Investigations*, vol. 6 (Baltimore: Helion, 1969), pp. 231–49.
20. Cf. *Theological Studies* 42 (1981): 109.
21. Sissela Bok, "Personal Directions for Care at the End of Life," *New England Journal of Medicine* 295 (1976): 367–69.
22. Joseph Sittler, *Grace Notes and Other Fragments* (Philadelphia: Fortress Press, 1981), p. 98.

23. Richard A. McCormick, S.J., *How Brave a New World* (New York: Doubleday, 1981), pp. 87–89.
24. Paul Ramsey, in *The Vatican Council and the World of Today* (Brown University, 1966), no pagination.
25. J. Francis Stafford, "The Year of the Family Revisited," *America* 144 (1981): 399–403.
26. Louis Janssens, "Artificial Insemination: Ethical Considerations" *Louvain Studies* 8 (1980): 3–29.
27. Ibid., p. 28.
28. Karl Rahner, "The Problem of Genetic Manifestation," *Theological Investigations*, vol. 9 (New York: Herder and Herder, 1972), p. 246.
29. Roger L. Shinn, "Homosexuality: Christian Conviction and Inquiry," in *The Same Sex*, ed. Ralph W. Weltge (Philadelphia: Pilgrim Press, 1969), pp. 43–54.
30. Ibid., p. 57.
31. Cf. note 10.
32. Shinn, op. cit., p. 51.
33. Ibid.
34. Cf. McCormick, *How Brave a New World?*, op. cit., pp. 197–98.
35. James F. Bresnahan, S.J., "Rahner's Christian Ethics," *America* 123 (1970): 351–54.
36. Ibid.
37. Gabriel Daly, "The Ultramontane Influence," *Tablet* 235 (1981): 392.
38. Roderick Mackenzie, S.J., "The Function of Scholars in Forming the Judgment of the Church," in *Theology of Renewal*, ed. L. K. Shook (Montreal: Palm Publishers, 1968), pp. 126–27.
39. Oswald von Nell-Breuning, S.J., "*Octogesimo anno,*" *Stimmen der Zeit* 187 (1971): 289–96.
40. *Catholic Review*, 4 March 1983, p. 1.
41. Bernard Häring, "Roman Catholic Directives," *Encyclopedia of Bioethics*, vol. 4 (New York: Free Press, 1978), pp. 1432–33.
42. *National Catholic Reporter*, 28 May 1969, p. 6.
43. Ibid.
44. *Documents*, p. 244.
45. *Documents*, p. 214.
46. Bernard Cooke, "The Responsibility of Theologians," *Commonweal* 107 (1980): 39–42.
47. Cf. note 2.
48. I have taken this citation from a release of *Documentary Service*, the former press department of the USCC.
49. B. C. Butler, "Authority and the Christian Conscience," *Clergy Review* 60 (1975): 3–17.
50. Bernard Häring, "Norms and Freedom in Contemporary Catholic Thought," a lecture delivered at Fordham University, 1975.
51. Juan Arzube, "When Is Dissent Legitimate?" *Catholic Journalist* (June 1978).
52. *Documents*, p. 48.
53. Karl Rahner, "Theologie und Lehramt," *Stimmen der Zeit* 198 (1980): 372.
54. André Naud, "Les Voix de l'église dans les questions morales," *Science et esprit*

32 (1980): 161–76. People often forget that when three of the conciliar bishops brought up the case of dissent and asked that it be clarified in *Lumen gentium*, the relator of the commission told the bishops that it is sufficient to consider the teaching of established theologians on the matter (*Acta Synodalia Sacrosancti Concilii Vaticani II*, 3: 8, 88). The teaching of established theologians, of course, has been that dissent is quite possible and legitimate.

Chapter 4/Justice in Health Care

1. Daniel Callahan, "Shattuck Lecture: Contemporary Biomedical Ethics," op. cit.
2. See President's Commission for the Study of Ethical Problems in Medicine and Biomedical and Behavioral Research, *Securing Access to Health Care* (Washington, D.C.: Government Printing Office, 1983). See also the Robert Wood Johnson Foundation's *Special Report* ("Updated Report on Access to Health Care for the American People" [1983]: n. 1).
3. Daniel Maguire, "The Primacy of Justice in Moral Theology," *Horizons* 10 (1983): 72–85.
4. John S. Cummins, "Oakland Statement on Women in Ministry," *Origins* 12 (1982): 331–33.
5. Victor Balke and Raymond Lucker, "Male and Female God Created Them," *Origins* 11 (1982): 333–38.
6. Matthew Clark, "American Catholic Women: Persistent Questions, Faithful Witness," *Origins* 12 (1982): 273–86.
7. *Catholic Chronicle*, 1 July 1983.
8. Cf. *Origins* 12 (1982): 286.
9. Ann Neale, "Health and Health Care Issues: Concerns for American Women," an address delivered 12 May 1980, Rayburn House Office Building.
10. Recently Stephen Colamero, M.D., Lorne A. Becker, M.D., and Michael Simpson, M.D., have contested many of the complaints about sex-role stereotyping. Cf. "Sex Bias in the Assessment of Patient Complaints," *Journal of Family Practice* 16 (1983): 1117–21.

Chapter 5/Sexuality

1. Peter Nichols, *The Pope's Divisions: The Roman Catholic Church Today* (London: Faber and Faber, 1981), p. 239.
2. Ibid.
3. *Documentation Catholique* 73 (1976): 181.
4. Roman Bleistein, S.J., "Kirchliche Autorität im Widerspruch," *Stimmen der Zeit* 101 (1976): 145–46.
5. "Sexualidad y moral cristiana," *Rázon y fe* 938 (March 1976): 198–201.
6. Alfons Auer et al., "Zweierlei Sexualethik," *Theologische Quartalschrift* 156 (1976): 148–58.
7. Bernard Häring, "Reflexionen zur Erklärung der Glaubenskongregation über

einige Fragen der Sexualethik," *Theologisch-Practische Quartalschrift* 124 (1976): 115–26.

8. I base this analysis on Louis Janssens, *Mariage et Fecondité* (Paris: Editions J. Duculot, 1967).

9. *De Genesi ad litteram* 9, c. 5, n. 9.

10. *De conjugiis adulterinis* 2, c. 12, n. 12.

11. *Summa Theologica* I–II, 94, a. 2.

12. *Acta Apostolicae Sedis* 22 (1930): 548.

13. *Documents*, pp. 250–55.

14. *Documents*, p. 253.

15. *Documents*, p. 250.

16. Louis Janssens, "Artificial Insemination: Ethical Considerations," *Louvain Studies* 8 (1980): 21. Many Catholic theologians agree with Janssens when he states that "it is also the Roman Theology which was at the root of *Humanae vitae* and the 'Declaration on Certain Questions Concerning Sexual Ethics,'" whereas the report of the Papal commission for the study of population, family and birth questions (1966) followed the personalist views of *Gaudium et spes*." In an interesting article, Joseph Ratzinger stated in 1971: "I should like to emphasize once more that I fully agree with Küng's distinction between Roman [-school] Theology and [Catholic] faith. I am convinced that Catholicism's survival depends on our ability to break out of the prison of the Roman-School Type." (J. Ratzinger, "Widersprüche im Buch von Hans Küng," in *Zum Problem Unfehlbarkeit*, ed. Karl Rahner [Freiburg, 1971]: 105).

17. F. Hürth, S.J., "La fécondation artificielle. Sa valeur morale et juridique," *Nouvelle revue théologique* 68 (1946): 413.

18. The paragraph numbers given refer to *De propagatione humanae prolis recte ordinanda* (Vatican City: Vatican Polyglot Press, 1968), a Latin version of *Humanae vitae*.

19. Cf. *Theological Studies* 29 (1968): 725.

20. Edward Genicot, S.J., *Institutiones Theologiae Moralis* (Brussels: L'Edition universelle, 1951) II, n. 664, p. 459.

21. John R. Quinn, "'New Context' for Contraception Teaching," *Origins* 10 (1980): 263–67.

22. G. Emmett Carter, "Spirit's Voice or Moral Decadence?" *Origins* 10 (1980): 276–77.

23. *On the Family* (Washington: USCC, 1981).

24. *Acta Apostolicae Sedis* 43 (1951): 845–46.

25. George Basil Hume, "Development of Marriage Teaching," *Origins* 10 (1980): 275–76.

26. Cf. McCormick, *How Brave a New World?*, op. cit., p. 260.

27. *On the Family*, op. cit., n. 32.

28. Johannes Gründel, "Zur Problematik der operativen Sterilisation in Katholischen Krankenhäusern," *Stimmen der Zeit* 199 (1981): 671–77.

29. John H. Wright, S.J., "An End to the Birth Control Controversy?" *America* 144 (1981): 175–78.

30. Cf. *Readings in Moral Theology*, vol. 1, pp. 72–73.

31. *Acta Apostolicae Sedis* 43 (1951): 835–36.

32. *Acta Apostolicae Sedis* 43 (1951): 850.

33. *Acta Apostolicae Sedis* 48 (1956): 470.

34. George Lobo, S.J., *Current Problems in Medical Ethics* (Allahabad: St. Paul Press, 1974), p. 152.

35. *The Pope Speaks* 21 (1976): 60–73.

36. Cf. "The Future of Woman in the Church," *Origins* 12 (1982): 1–9.

37. Cf. *Documentation catholique* 76 (1979): 715–22.

38. Cf. Richard A. McCormick, S.J., *Notes on Moral Theology 1965–1980* (Lanham, MD: University Press of America, 1981), p. 838.

39. *On the Family*, op. cit., n. 84.

40. "Le problème pastoral des chrétiens divorcés et remariés," *Vie spirituelle: supplement* 109 (May 1974): 145.

41. Cited in Philip S. Kaufman, "An Immoral Morality?" *Commonweal* 107 (1980): 493–97.

42. Cited in Bernard Häring, "Pastorale Erwägungen zur Bischofssynode über Familie und Ehe," *Theologie der Gegenwart* 24 (1981): 71–80.

Chapter 6/Dignity, Passages, Madness, Suffering, Dying

1. *Documents*, p. 227.

2. Joseph A. Califano, *The 1982 Report on Drug Abuses and Alcoholism* (New York: Warner Books, 1982), pp. 27–28.

3. Thomas E. Clarke, S.J., "Public Policy and Christian Discernment," in *Personal Values in Public Policy*, ed. John Haughey (Ramsey, NJ: Paulist, 1979), pp. 212–31.

4. J. H. van den Berg, *The Psychology of the Sickbed* (Pittsburgh: Duquesne University Press, 1966), p. 37.

5. Renee C. Fox, *Experiment Perilous* (Philadephia: University of Pennslyvania Press, 1959), p. 115.

6. Alexander Solzhenitsyn, *Cancer Ward* (New York: Bantam Books, 1969), p. 54.

7. Ibid., p. 446.

8. *Experiment Perilous*, op. cit., p. 119.

9. *Superintendent of Belchertown State School v. Saikewicz*, 370 N. E. Rep., 2d. sec., 417–35 (Mass., 1977).

10. *Washington Post*, 18 February 1978.

11. George Annas, "The Incompetent's Right to Die: The Case of Joseph Saikewicz," *Hastings Center Report* 8 (Feb., 1978) 21–23.

12. Cf. Richard A. McCormick, S.J., *How Brave a New World?* (New York: Doubleday, 1981), p. 373.

13. Edmund N. Santurri and William Werpehowski, "Substituted Judgment and the Terminally-Ill Incompetent," *Thought* 57 (1982): 484–501.

14. Edmund D. Pellegrino, M.D., "No Code Orders: Medical Crisis, Medical Choice and Patient Good," forthcoming.

15. This is Pellegrino's phrase.

16. Michel Quoist, *Prayers* (New York: Avon Books, 1975), pp. 84–86.

17. *Documents*, p. 161.

18. Joseph Kern, S.J., *De Sacramento E. Unctionis* (Ratisbon: Pustet, 1907).
19. P. Anciaux, *Collectania Mechliniensia* 44 (1959): 7–21.
20. John R. Connery, S.J., "Notes on Moral Theology," *Theological Studies* 20 (1959): 618.
21. *New Catholic Encyclopedia*, vol. 4 (New York: McGraw-Hill, 1967), p. 689.
22. Ibid.
23. 2 Corinthians 5:10.
24. Bruno Schüller, S.J., "Todsünde—Sünde zum Tod?" *Theologie und Philosophie* 42 (1967): 321–40.
25. *New Catholic Encyclopedia*, vol. 4, op. cit., p. 694.
26. John R. Connery, S.J., *Abortion: The Development of the Roman Catholic Perspective* (Chicago: Loyola University Press, 1977).
27. John Noonan, "An Almost Absolute Value in History," in *The Morality of Abortion*, ed. John Noonan (Cambridge: Harvard University Press, 1970), pp. 1–59.
28. André E. Hellegers, "Amazing Historical and Biological Errors in Abortion Decision," *Hospital Progress* 54 (May 1973): 16–17.
29. *Documents*, p. 256.
30. Pope Paul VI, "Pourquois L'Eglise ne peut accepter l'avortement," *Documentation catholique*, 70 (1973): 4–5.
31. Ibid.
32. "Déclaration des Évêques belges sur l'avortement," *Documentation catholique*, 20 (1973): 432–38.
33. Ibid., p. 434.
34. "Déclaration des Évêques suisses sur l'avortement," *Documentation catholique*, 70 (1973): 381.
35. "Déclaration des Évêques du Québec," *Documentation catholique*, 20 (1973): 382–84.
36. "Le problème de l'avortement: Lettre pastorale des Évêques Allemands," *Documentation catholique* 70 (1973): 626–29.
37. Ibid., p. 628.
38. "'Fristenregelung' Entshieden abgelehnt," *Ruhrwort* (8 Dec. 1973): 6.
39. "Déclaration du Conseil permanent de l'Episcopat français sur l'avortement," *Documentation catholique*, 70 (1973): 676–79.
40. NCCB pastoral message, 83.
41. Michael J. Walsh, S.J., "What the Bishops Say" *Month* 234 (1973): 172–75.
42. Ph. Delhaye, "Le magistère catholique et l'avortement," *Esprit et vie* 83 (1973): 449–57.
43. Walsh, op. cit., p. 174.
44. Ibid., pp. 173–74.
45. "A New Catholic Strategy on Abortion" *Month* 234 (1973): 169–70.
46. Karl Rahner, "Basic Observations on the Subject of Changeable and Unchangeable Factors in the Church," *Theological Investigations*, vol. 14 (New York: Seabury, 1976), pp. 3–23.
47. "Declaration on Euthanasia," 443.
48. Albert C. Outler, "The Beginnings of Personhood: Theoiogical Considerations," *Perkins Journal* 27 (1973): 28–34.
49. Denis O'Callaghan, "Moral Principle and Exception," *Furrow* 22 (1971): 686–96.

50. Susan Teft Nicholson, *Abortion and the Roman Catholic Church* (Knoxville: Religious Ethics, 1979).
51. Cf. note 48.
52. Rahner, *Theological Investigations*, vol. 9, pp., 226, 236.
53. Bernard Häring, *Medical Ethics* (Notre Dame: Fides, 1973), pp. 81ff.
54. *Hospital Progress* 54 (March 1973): 83.
55. Paul Micallef, "Abortion and the Principles of Legislation," *Laval théologique et philosophique* 28 (1972): 267–303.
56. John Courtney Murray, *We Hold These Truths* (New York: Sheed and Ward, 1960), pp. 166–67.
57. *Catholic Standard*, 6 April 1978.
58. Daniel Callahan, "Abortion: Thinking and Experiencing," *Christianity and Crisis* 32 (1973): 295–98.
59. *America*, 28 May 1983, 409.
60. *America*, 2 July 1983, 20.
61. *Catholic Chronicle*, 1 July 1983, 1.
62. *Inside Passage*, 8 Oct. 1982, 4–5.
63. Kevin O'Rourke and Benedict Ashley, *Health Care Ethics* (St. Louis: Catholic Hospital Association, 1977), p. 323.
64. Ibid., p. 324.
65. For this debate, cf. *How Brave a New World?*, 87–98.
66. *How Brave a New World?*, 99–116.
67. *An Ethical Evaluation of Fetal Experimentation* (St. Louis: Pope John XXIII Center, 1976), pp. 75–76.
68. *Journal of the American Medical Association* 227 (1974): 728.
69. "Declaration on Euthanasia," 10.
70. *Hastings Report* 12 (August 1982): 6.
71. Norman Frost, M.D., "Putting Hospitals on Notice" *Hastings Report* 12 (August 1983): 5–8.
72. "Declaration on Euthanasia," 5.
73. This is available as a brochure from the United States Catholic Conference.
74. Cf. Ambrogio Valsecchi, *Controversy* (Washington, D.C.: Corpus, 1968).
75. *Acta Apostolicae Sedis* 43 (1951): 845–46.
76. Victorina Peralta, "Challenge of Aging for the Church," *New Catholic World* 223 (1980): 105–8.
77. Drew Christiansen, S.J., "The Elderly and Their Families: The Problems of Dependence," *New Catholic World* 223 (1980): 100–4.
78. Ibid., p. 102.
79. Ibid., p. 104.
80. Cited in Christiansen, op. cit., p. 104.

Afterword

Project Ten is the realization of the dreams of many people that the springs of religious faith might flow more freely into the parched regions of human health care. It seems strange that the outflow has dwindled to a mere trickle. After all, the phenomenon of healers, the very notions of therapy or salvation, and the arts of caring had their origins in religious experience. But the disjunction has occurred. When contemporary writers address various moral issues of medical ethics—genetics, transplantation, cessation of treatment, care for handicapped newborns, care of the dying—they do so in legal, economic, and philosophical, not theological, terms. Ironically, the deepest experiences of patients, families, and professionals, when faced with issues of healing and suffering, birth and death, continue to be framed in profound languages of hope and guilt, fidelity and sin, justice and responsibility, not in languages of utilitarianism, deontology, or cost-benefit analysis. In life and death crises persons reach into those deep reservoirs of belief and value that we call faith traditions. People respond to decisions of health care, at least in part, in terms of the ethics of their belief communities, that is, Judaism, Christianity, Islam, Hinduism, and the other world views and faiths. When health professionals seek to understand the patient, we think it is much more important to know whether she is a Jehovah's Witness, Orthodox Jew, or devout Roman Catholic than whether she is a deontologist, situationalist, capitalist, or socialist.

The programs of Project Ten seek to reclaim our awareness of the religious heritages of health-beliefs and values. We do this through publications like our current series of volumes on health and medicine in specific faith traditions, one of which is this fine volume by Richard McCormick. A forthcoming two-volume historical set on religion and medicine will present this treasury of wisdom in an encyclopedic format. Ahead are an ambitious clinical phase and a more permanent institutional form for this project.

We will sponsor a wide spectrum of clinical projects to investigate the inter-actions of faith orientations with health-care decisions. Cessation of treat-ment, human experimentation, genetic counseling are examples of issues to be carefully explored. Insights from these clinical studies will be shared with the public through publications and other media presentations. We hope to invest in the training of a new generation of more spiritually and morally sensitive doctors, nurses, and other health professionals.

Project Ten is funded by the Lutheran General Health Care System and the Lutheran Institute of Human Ecology. To reach its fullest potential it needs support from benefactors in hospitals, churches, and other sectors. Under Lutheran Institute of Human Ecology President George B. Caldwell, M.H.A., the project is guided by Kenneth L. Vaux, Dr.Theol., a theolo-gican/ethicist at the Health Science Center of the University of Illinois at Chicago, and by Martin E. Marty, Ph.D., Fairfax M. Cone Distinguished Service Professor at the University of Chicago. David T. Stein, Ph.D., project administrator, and James P. Wind, Ph.D., director of research, constitute the full-time operational staff. A management team consisting of Lawrence E. Holst, S.T.M., chief of Pastoral Care (chair); L. James Wylie, B.Th., vice president; Richard R. Short, Ed.D., vice president, Education and Research; Patrick R. Staunton, M.D., chief of Psychiatry; and William G. Bartholome, M.D., medical ethicist/ambulatory pedia-trics, give ongoing oversight to the project. A distinguished international advisory board of scholars and experts provides sustaining counsel to the project. Currently these members are: Darrel W. Amundsen, Ph.D., Bell-ingham, Washington; Glen W. Davidson, Ph.D., Springfield, Illinois; Prakosh Desai, M.D., River Forest, Illinois; H. Tristram Engelhardt, Jr., Ph.D., M.D., Houston, Texas; Daniel W. Foster, M.D., Dallas, Texas; Karen A. Lebacqz, Ph.D., Berkeley, California; F. Dean Lueking, Ph.D., River Forest, Illinois; Richard A. McCormick, S.J., S.T.D., Washington, D.C.; Ronald L. Numbers, Ph.D., Madison, Wisconsin; Fazlur Rahman, Ph.D., Chicago, Illinois; Dietrich Ritschl, Ph.D., Heidelberg, Germany; Mary-Carroll Sullivan, R.N., M.T.S., Boston, Massachusetts, and Ernst L. Wynder, M.D., New York, New York. We invite the inquiries and ex-pressions of support from any and all who seek to invigorate the spiritual and moral vitality of the health-care enterprise as well as from those con-cerned with renewing the contributions of religious bodies to this range of questions.

KENNETH L. VAUX